Vive Le Color!

ENERGY
COLORING BOOK & PENCILS

ABRAMS NOTERIE, NEW YORK

ABRAMS
THE ART OF BOOKS SINCE 1949

115 West 18th Street
New York, NY 10011
www.abramsbooks.com

Abrams Noterie products are available at special discounts when purchased in quantity for premiums and promotions as well as fundraising or educational use. Special editions can also be created to specification. For details, contact specialsales@abramsbooks.com or the address below.

Printed and bound in China
10 9 8 7 6 5 4

Published in 2015 by Abrams Noterie, an imprint of ABRAMS. All rights reserved. No portion of this book may be reproduced, stored in a retrieval system, or transmitted in any form or by any means, mechanical, electronic, photocopying, recording, or otherwise, without written permission from the publisher.

English translation copyright © 2015 Abrams Noterie

Copyright © 2015 Hachette Livre (Marabout)
Illustrations © Shutterstock
Design: Else

ISBN: 978-1-4197-2052-9

Check out the full line of *Viue Le Color!* coloring books at www.abramsnoterie.com

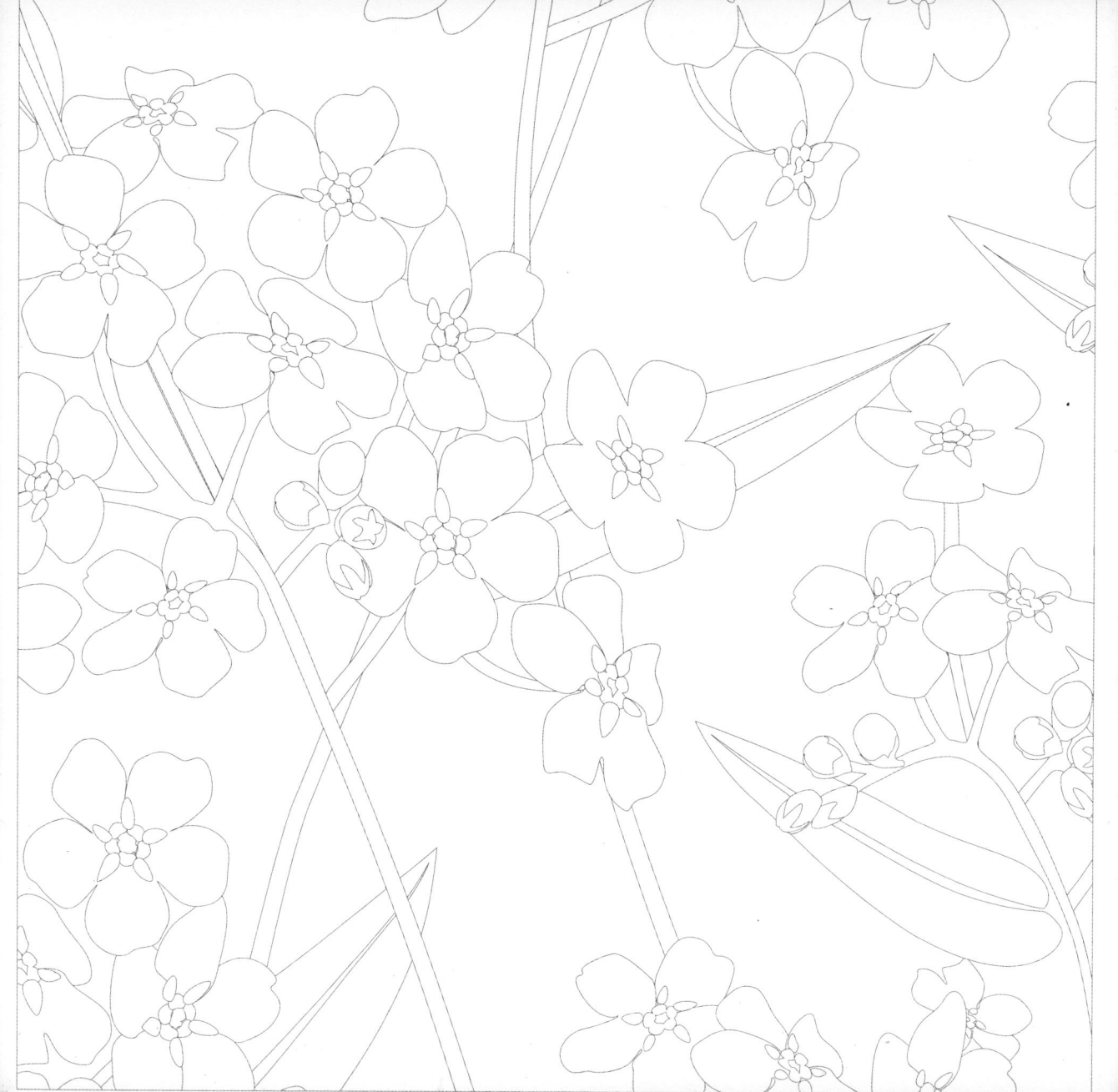

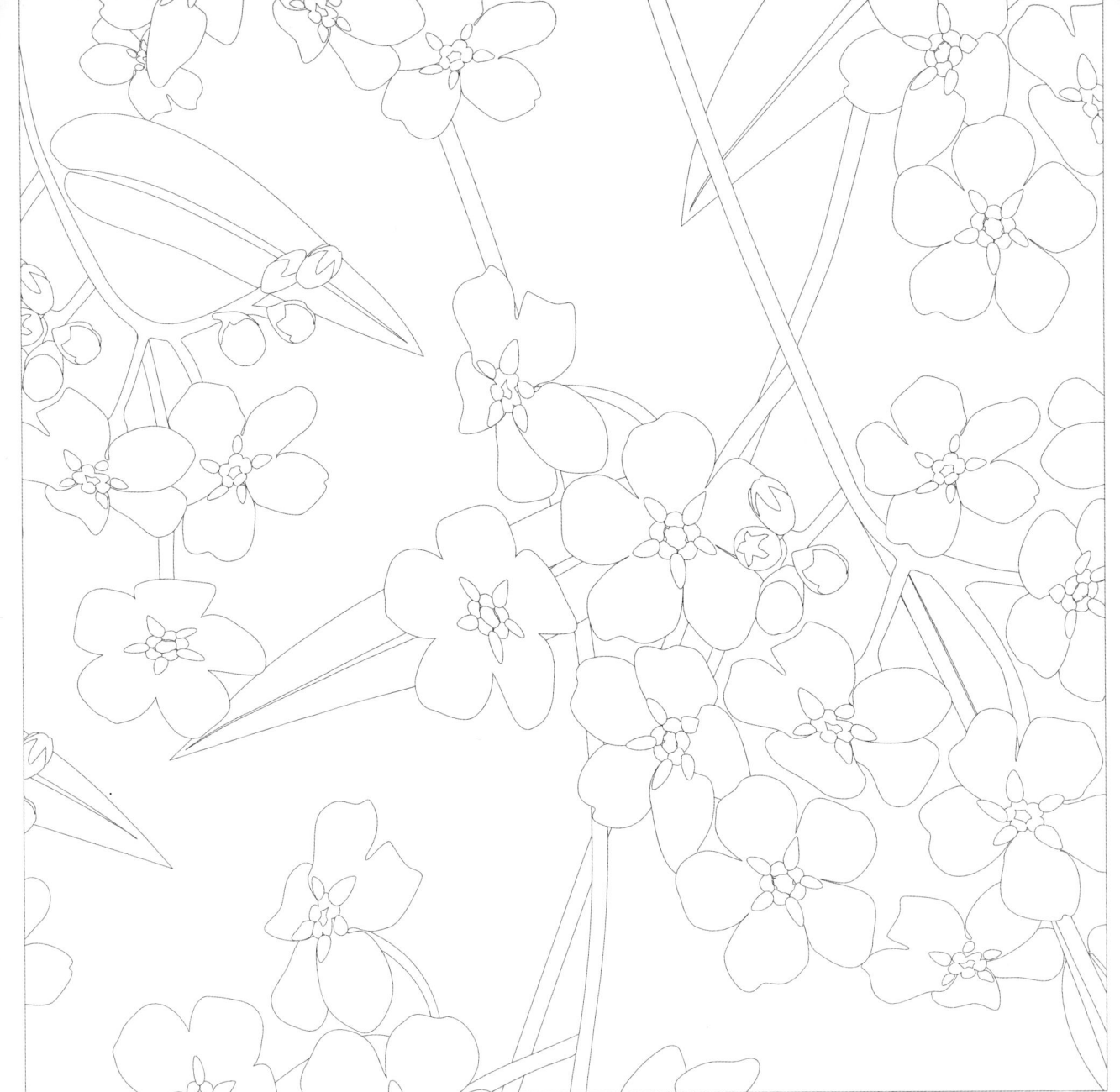

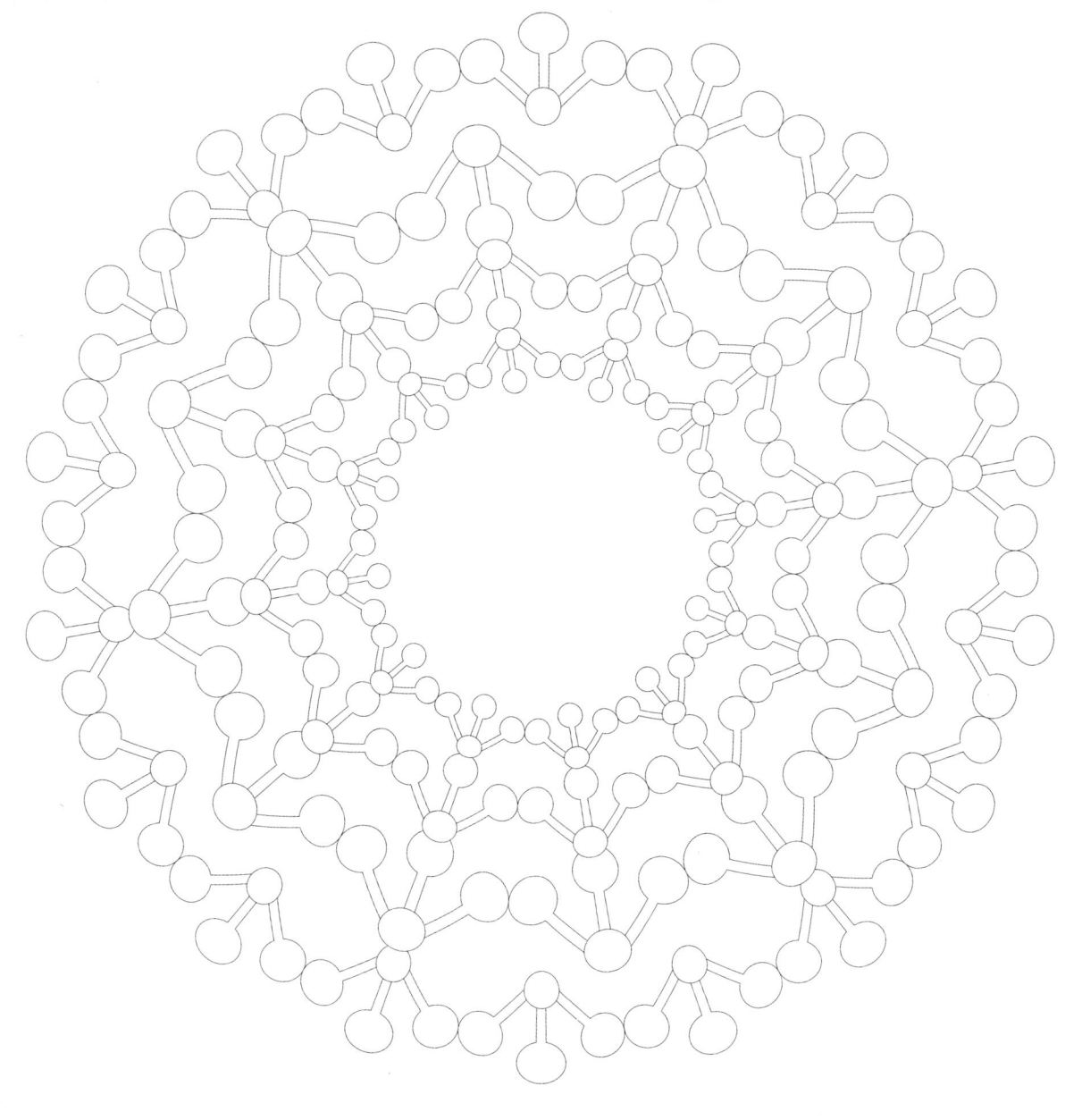

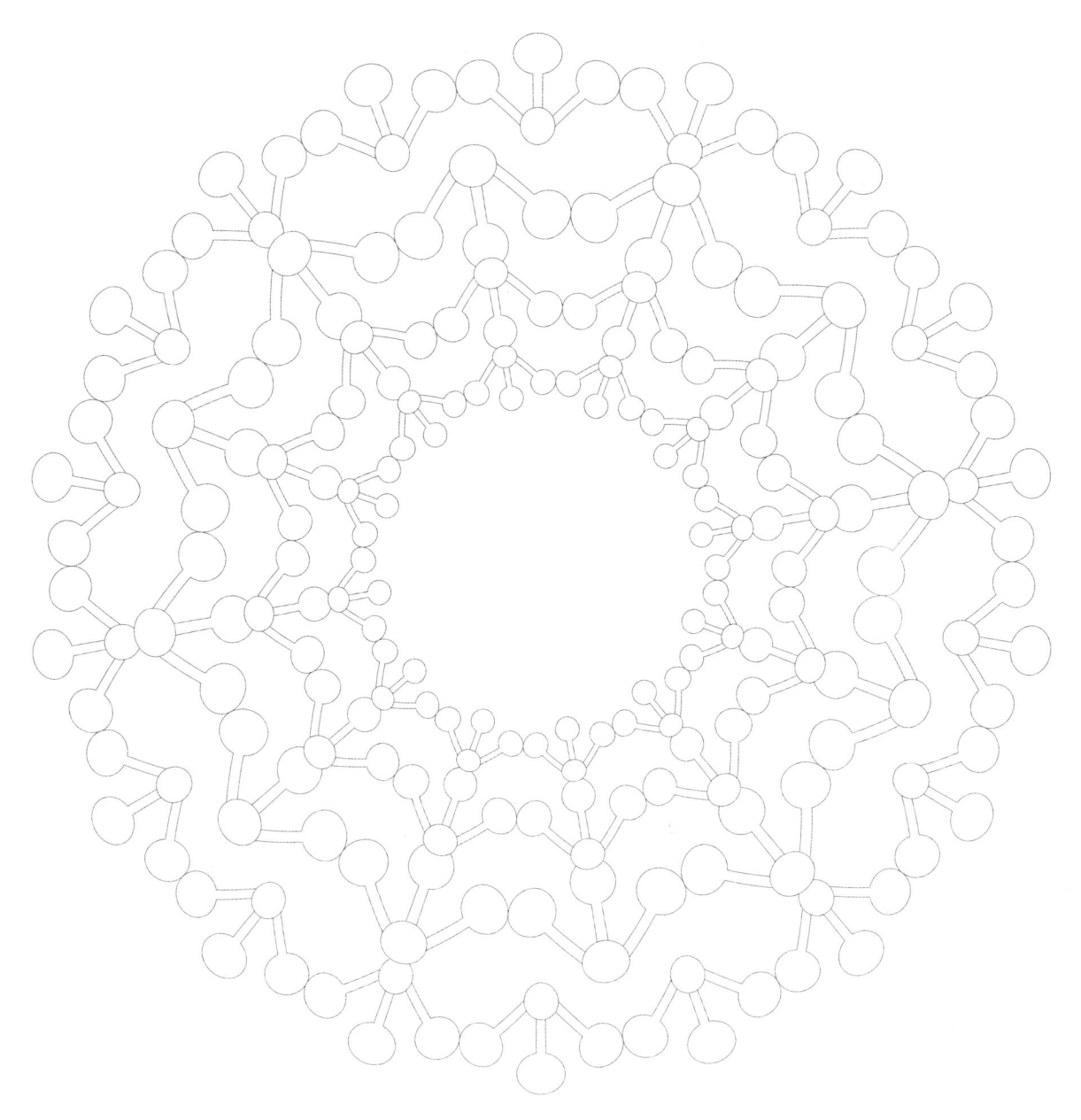

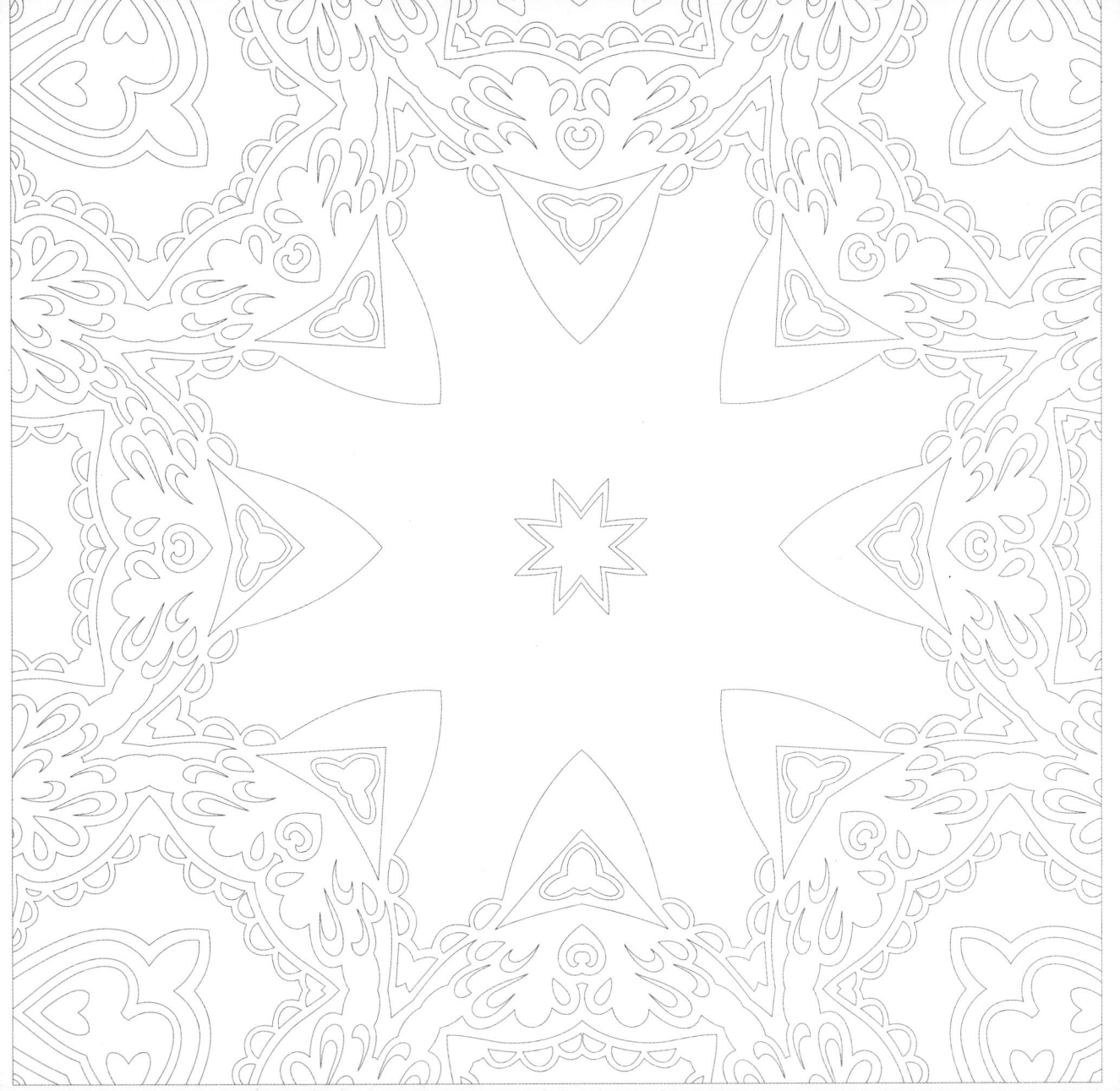

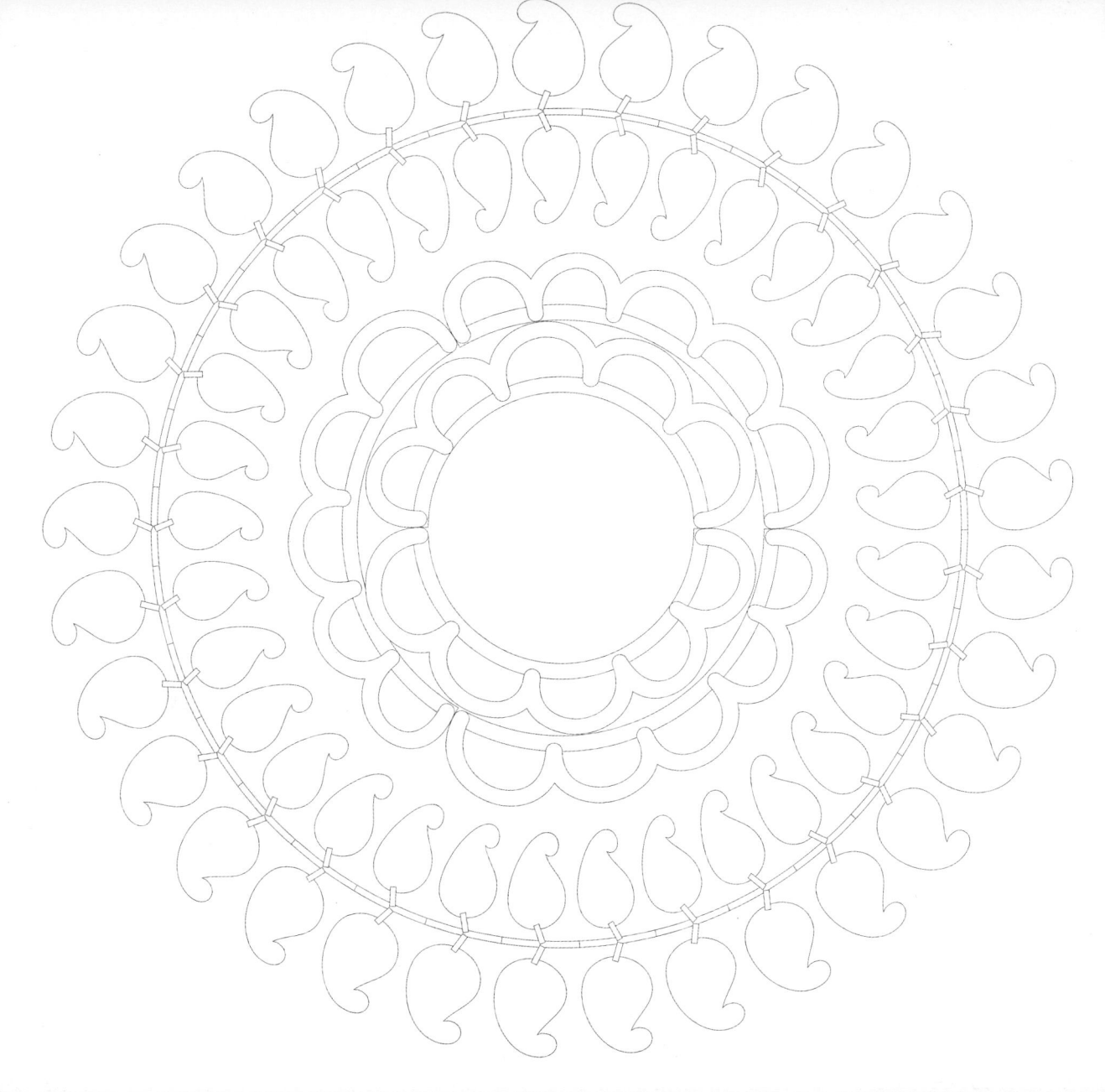

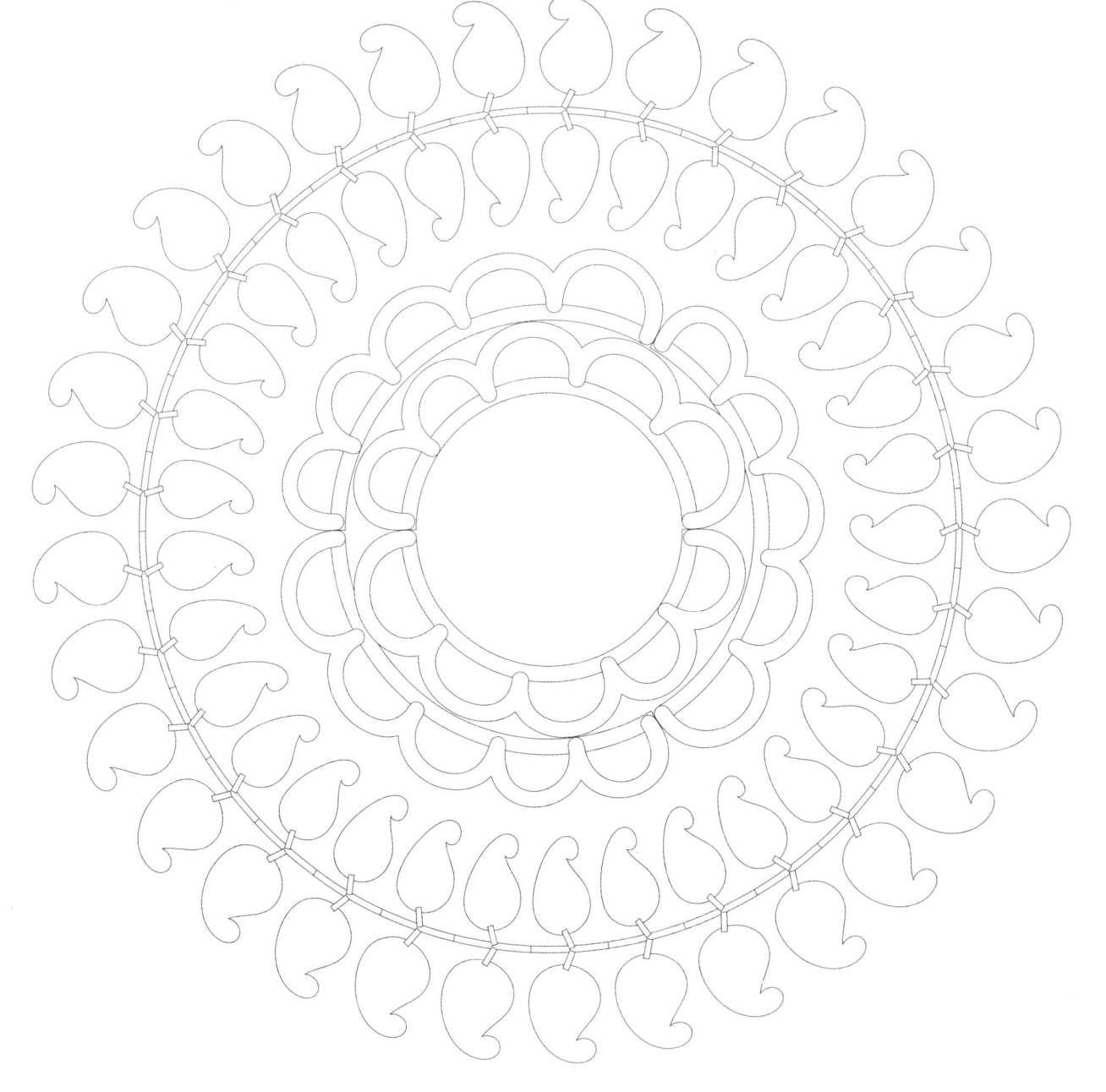

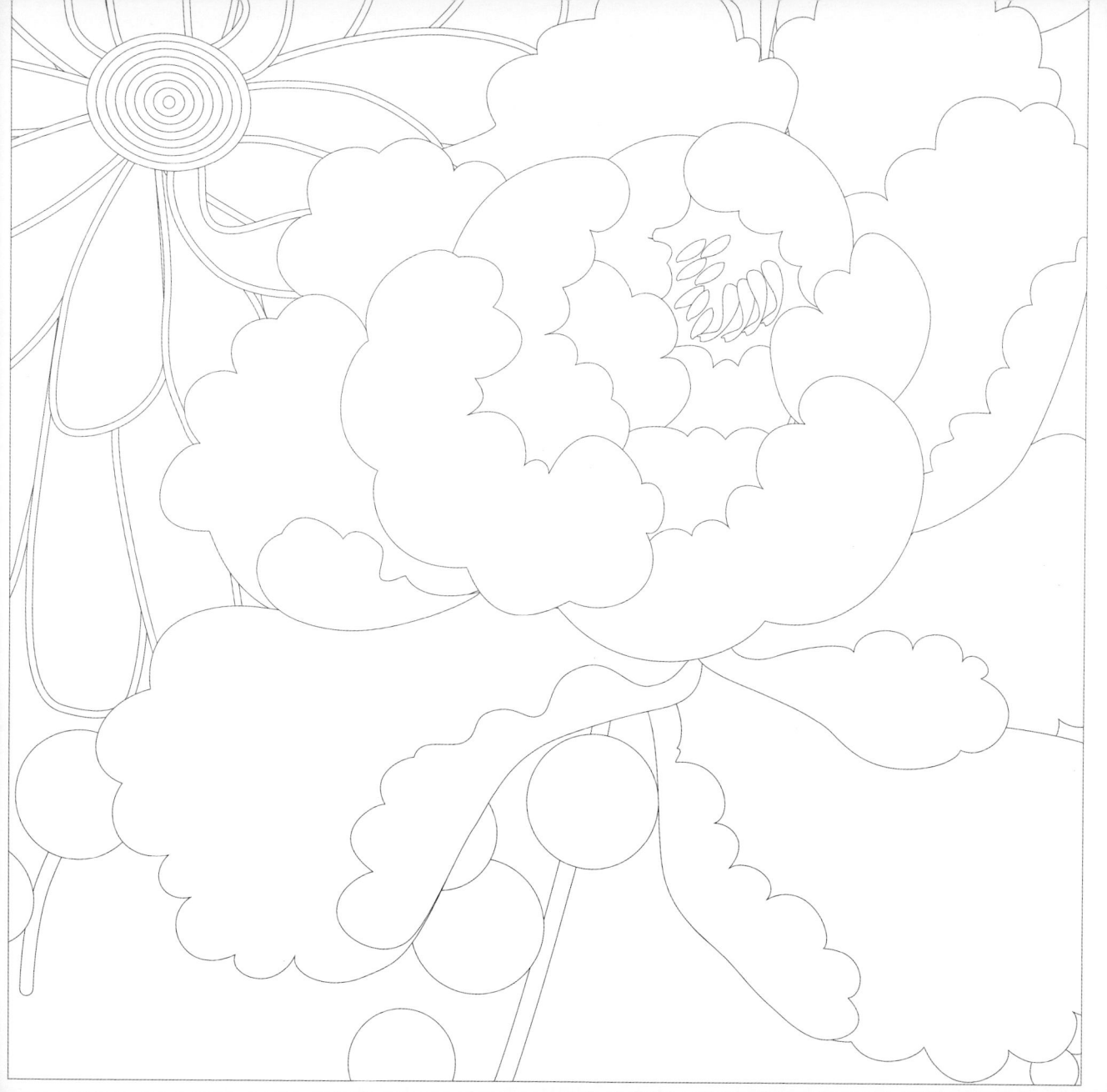

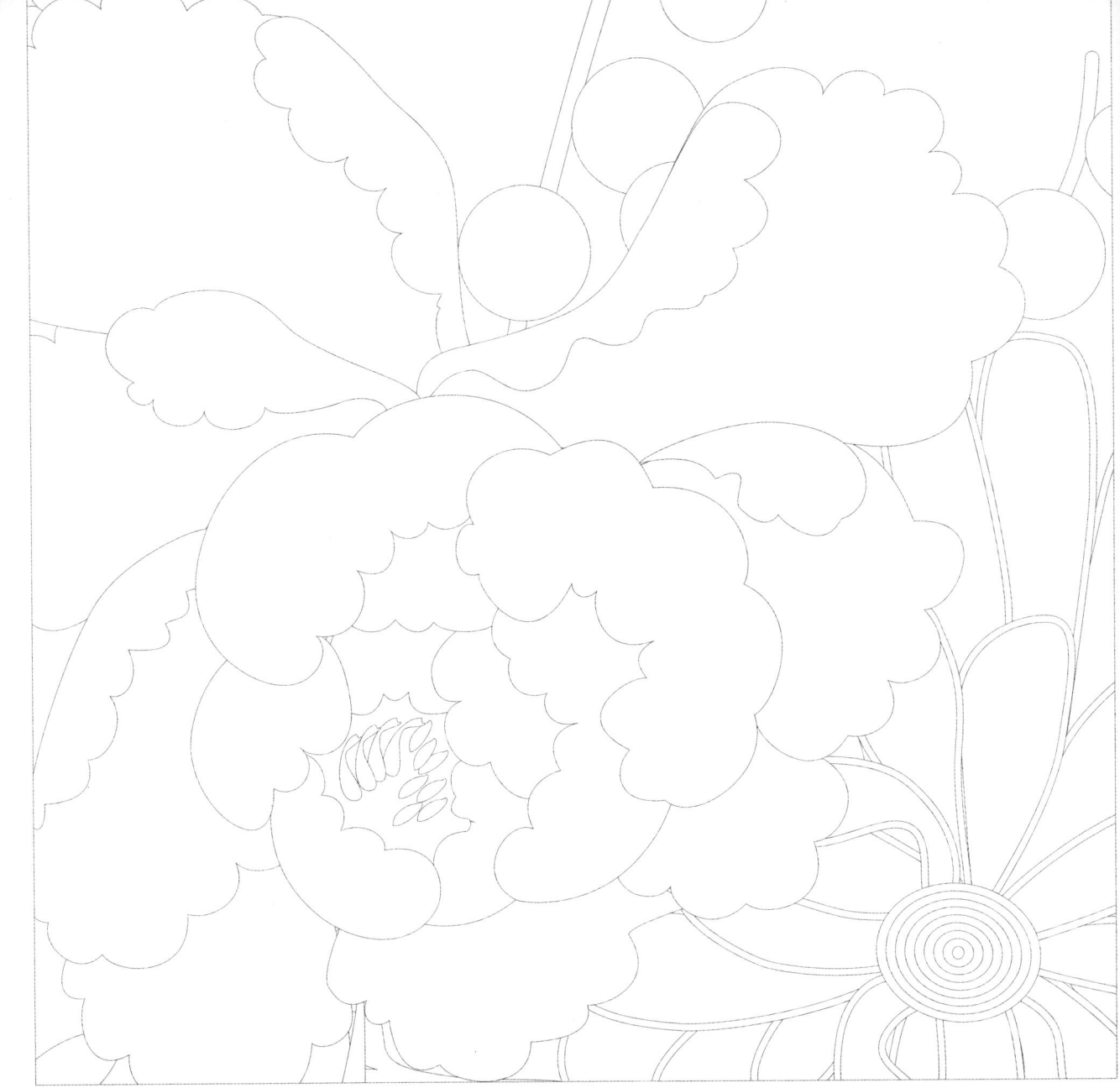

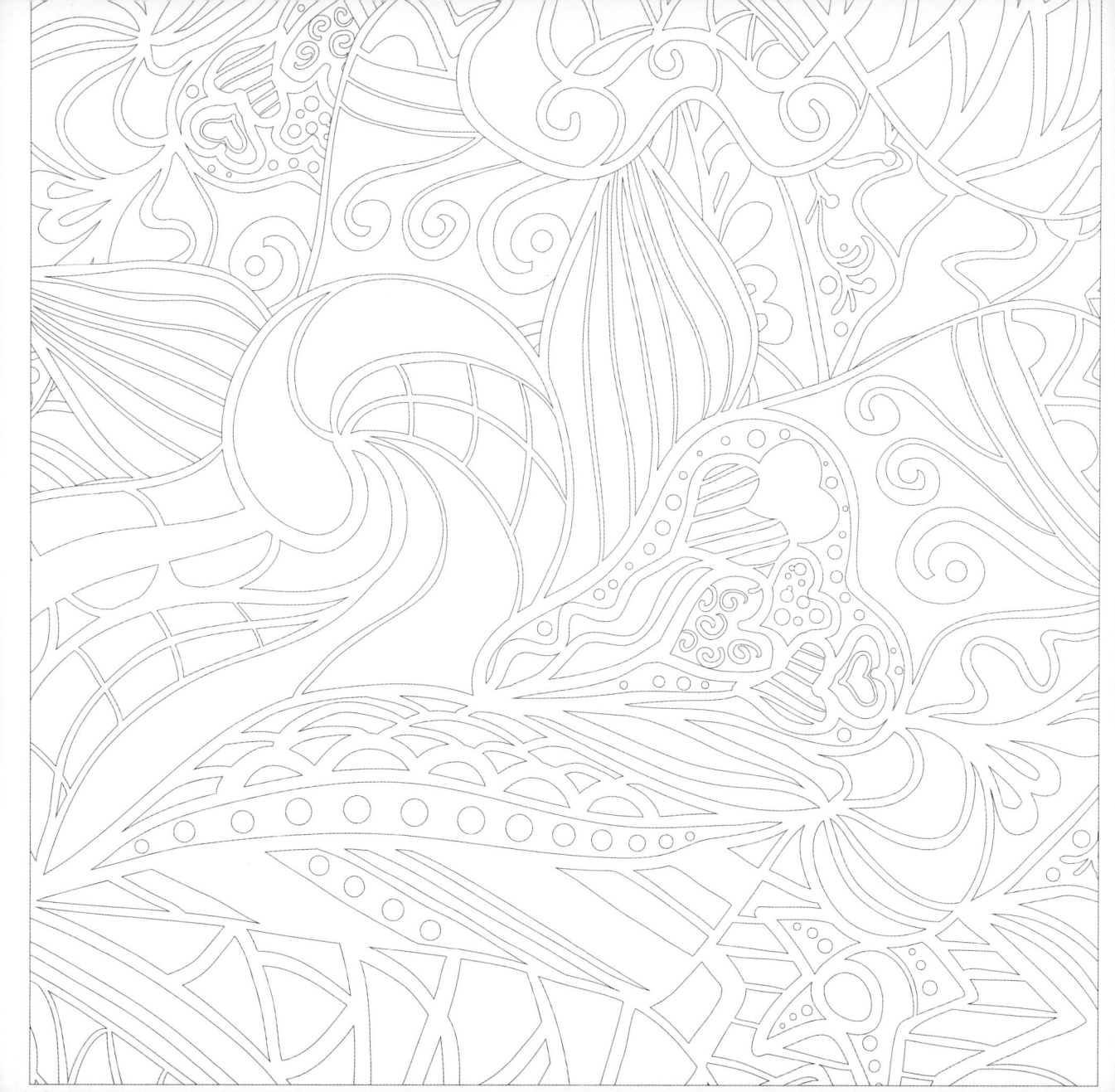

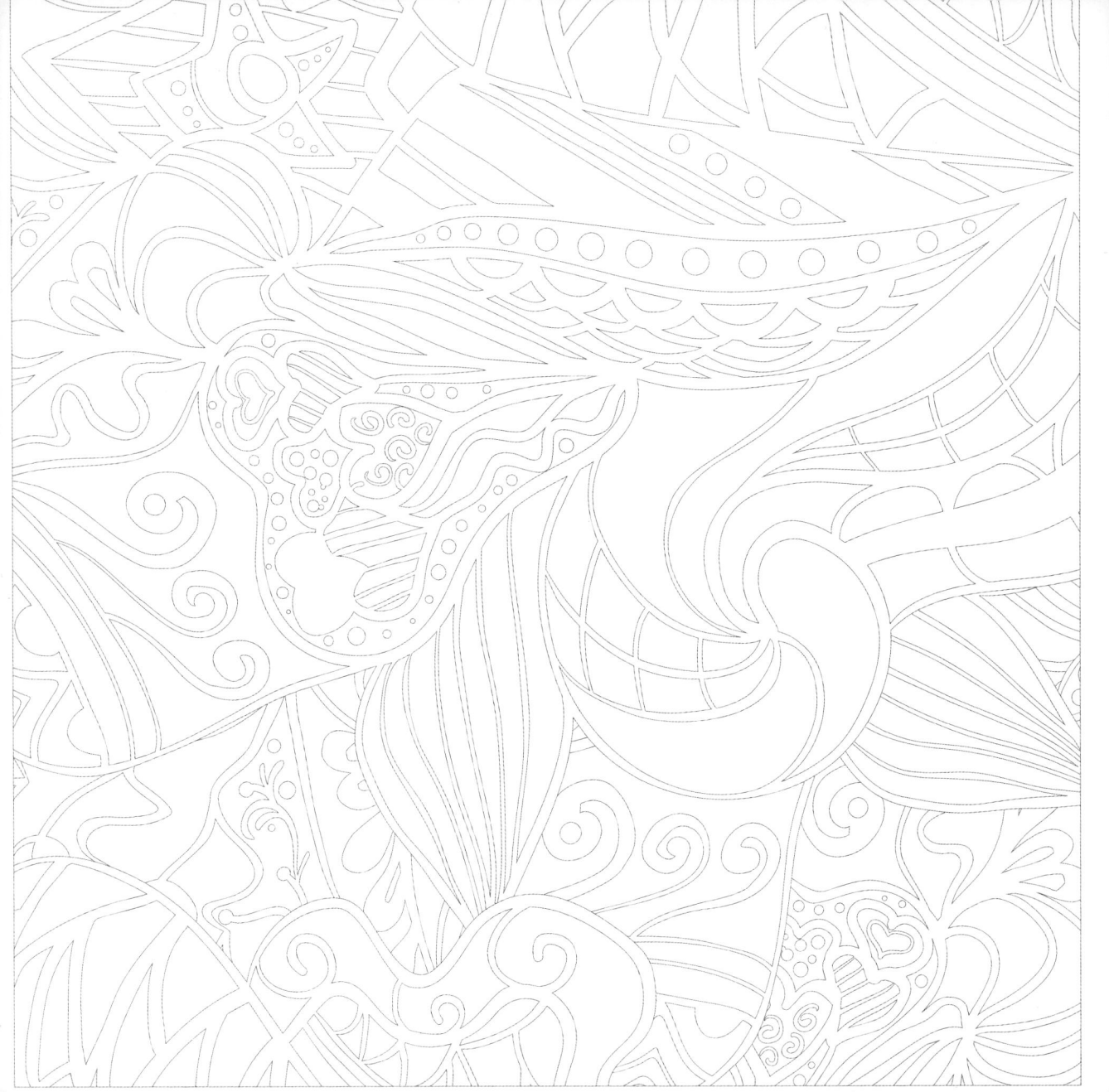

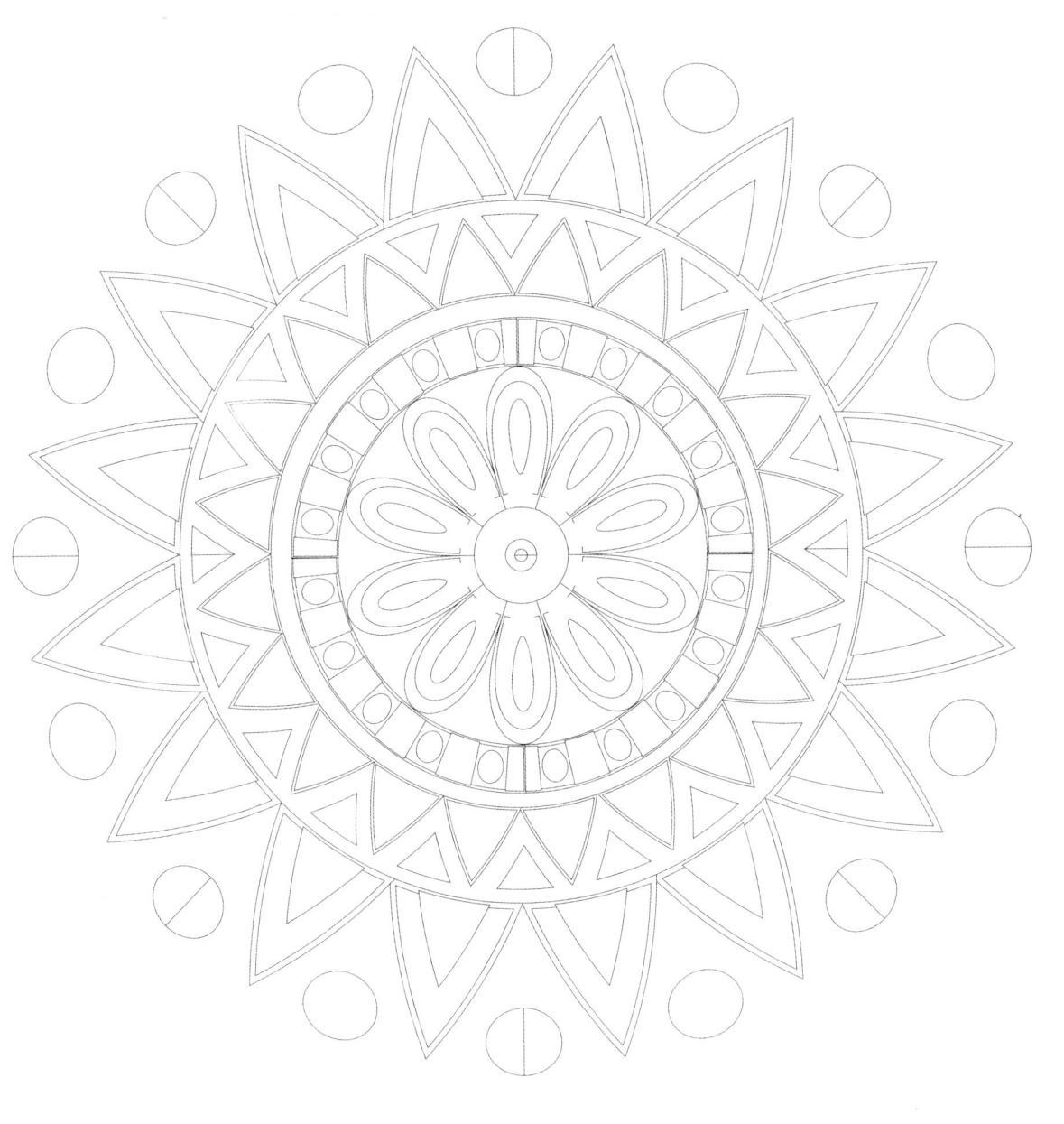

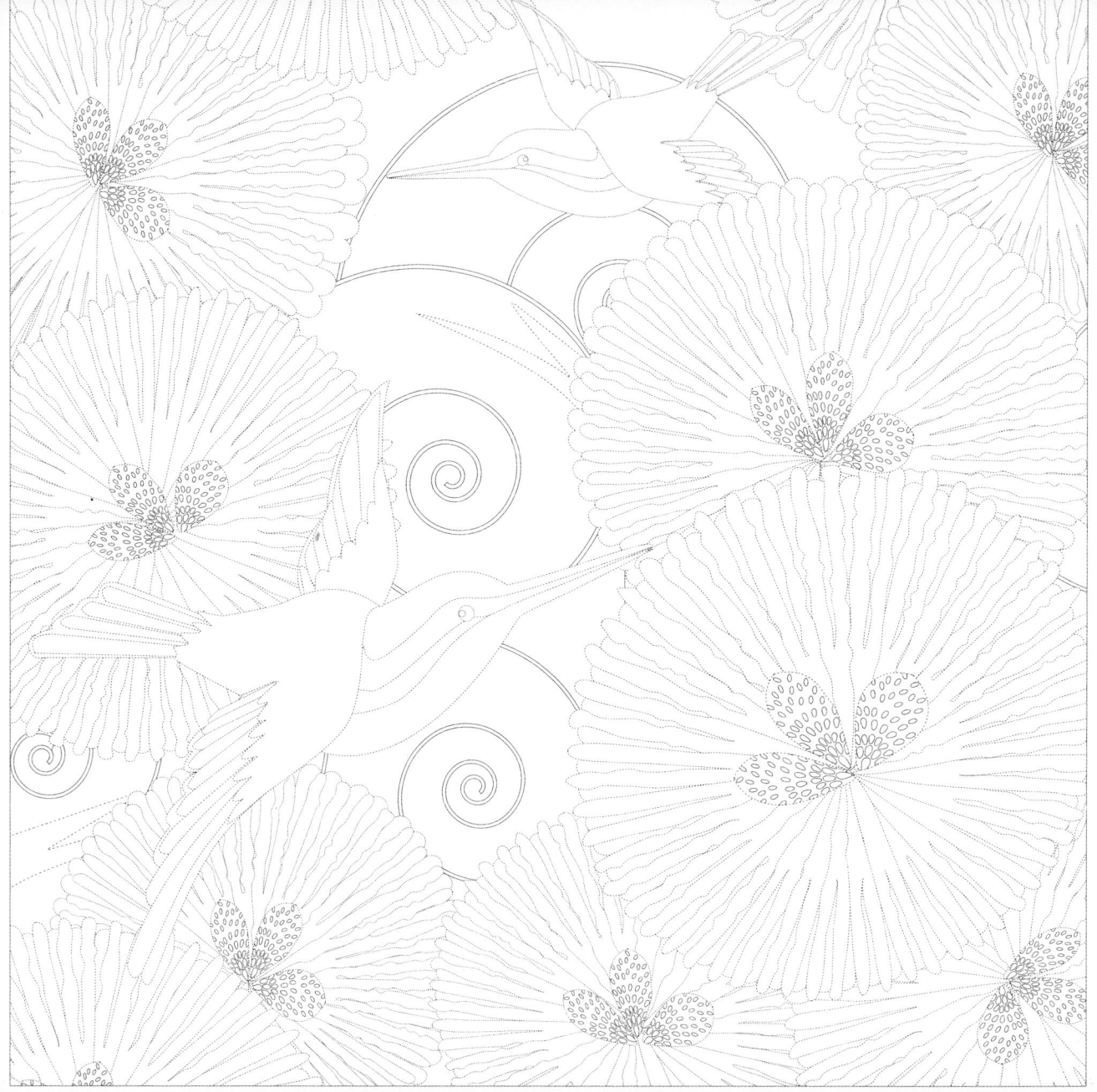

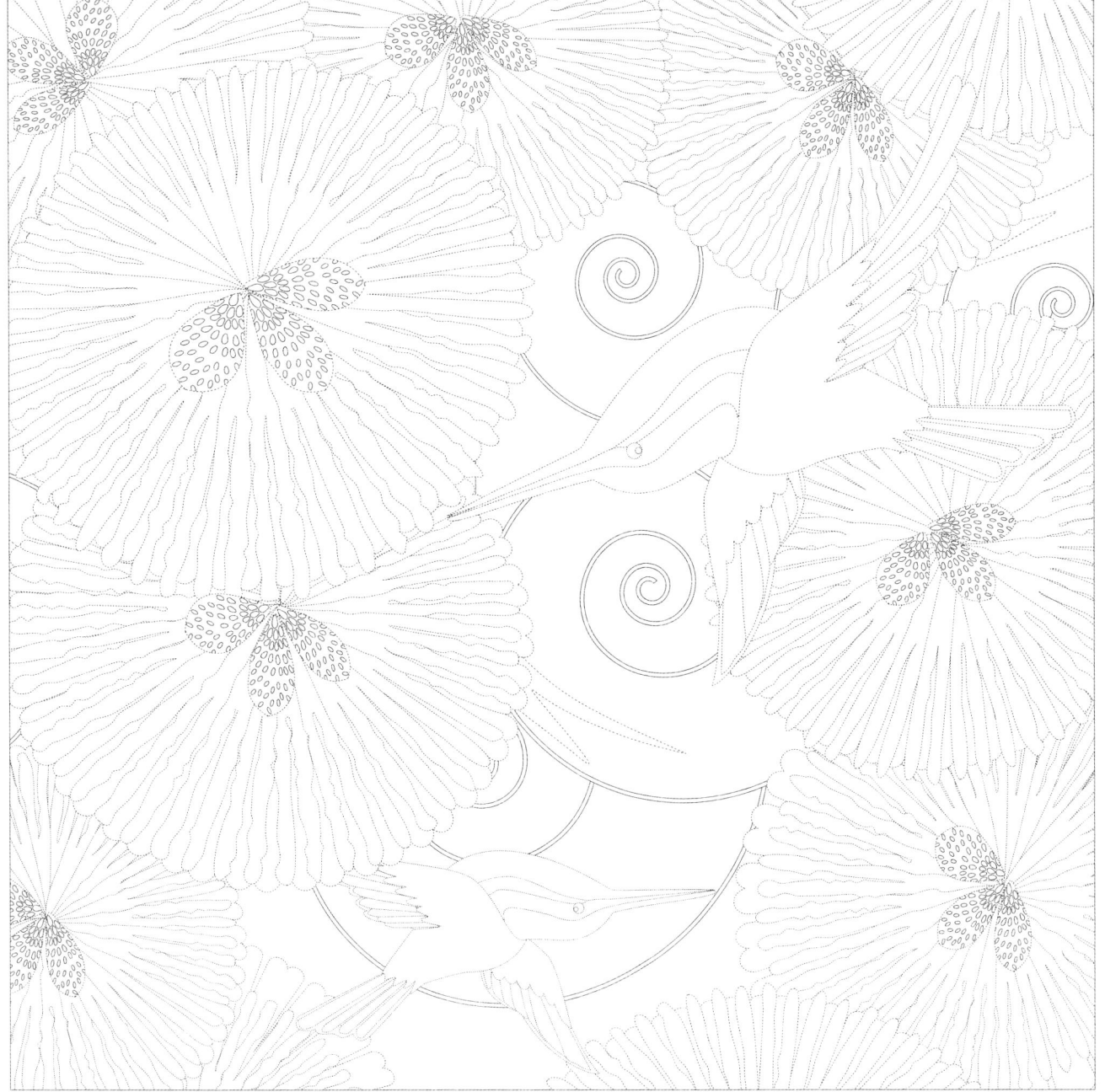

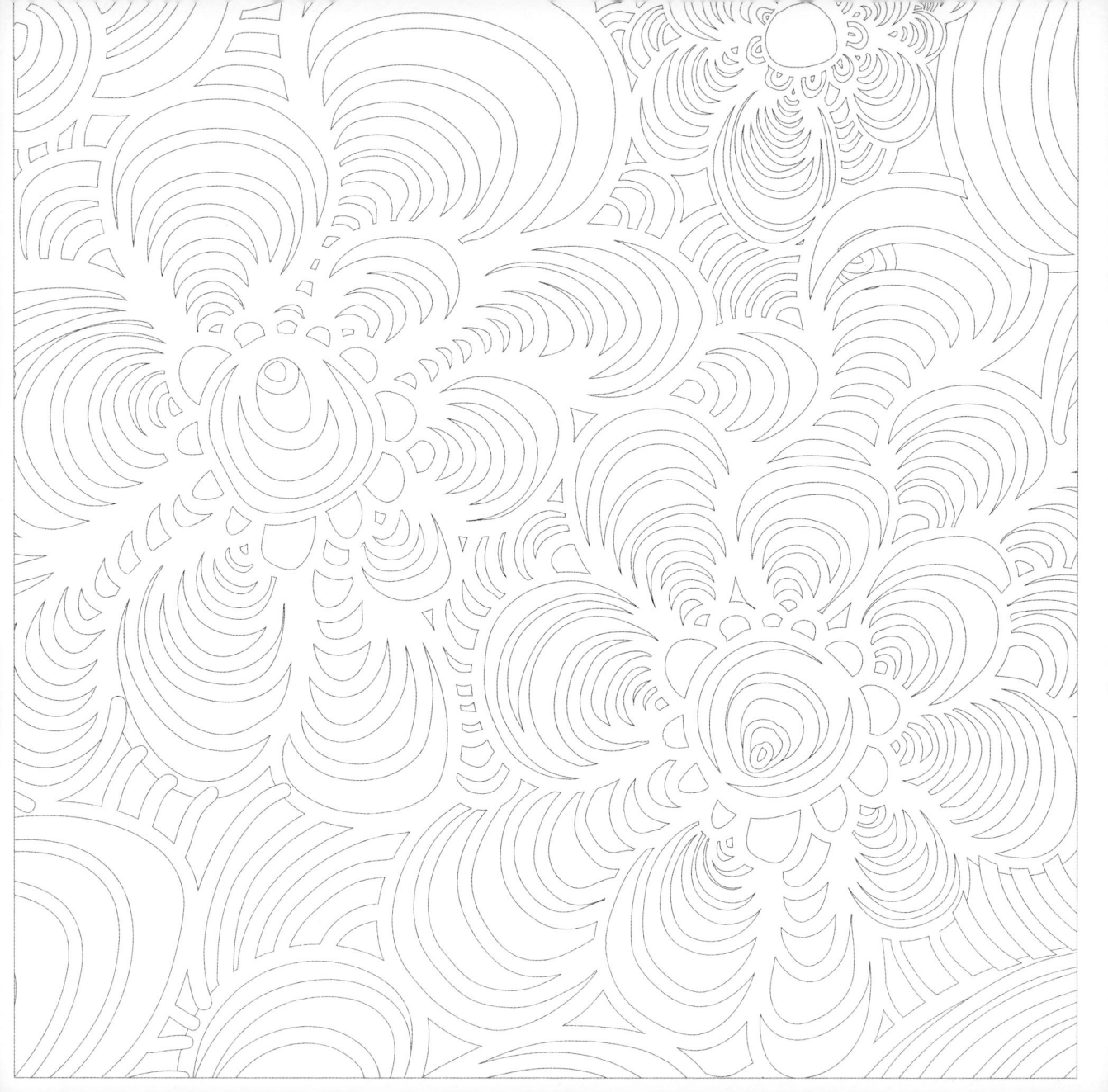

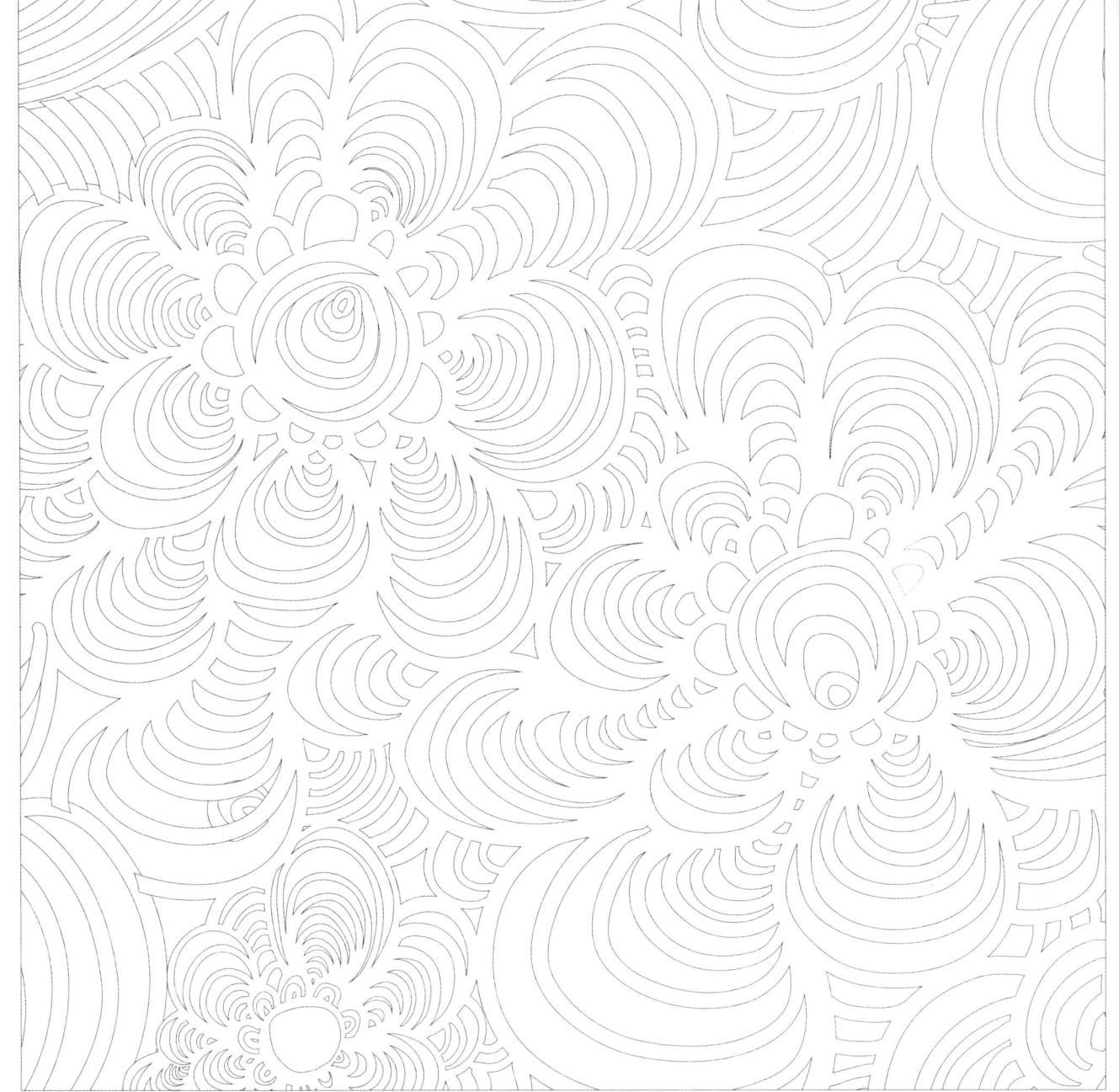

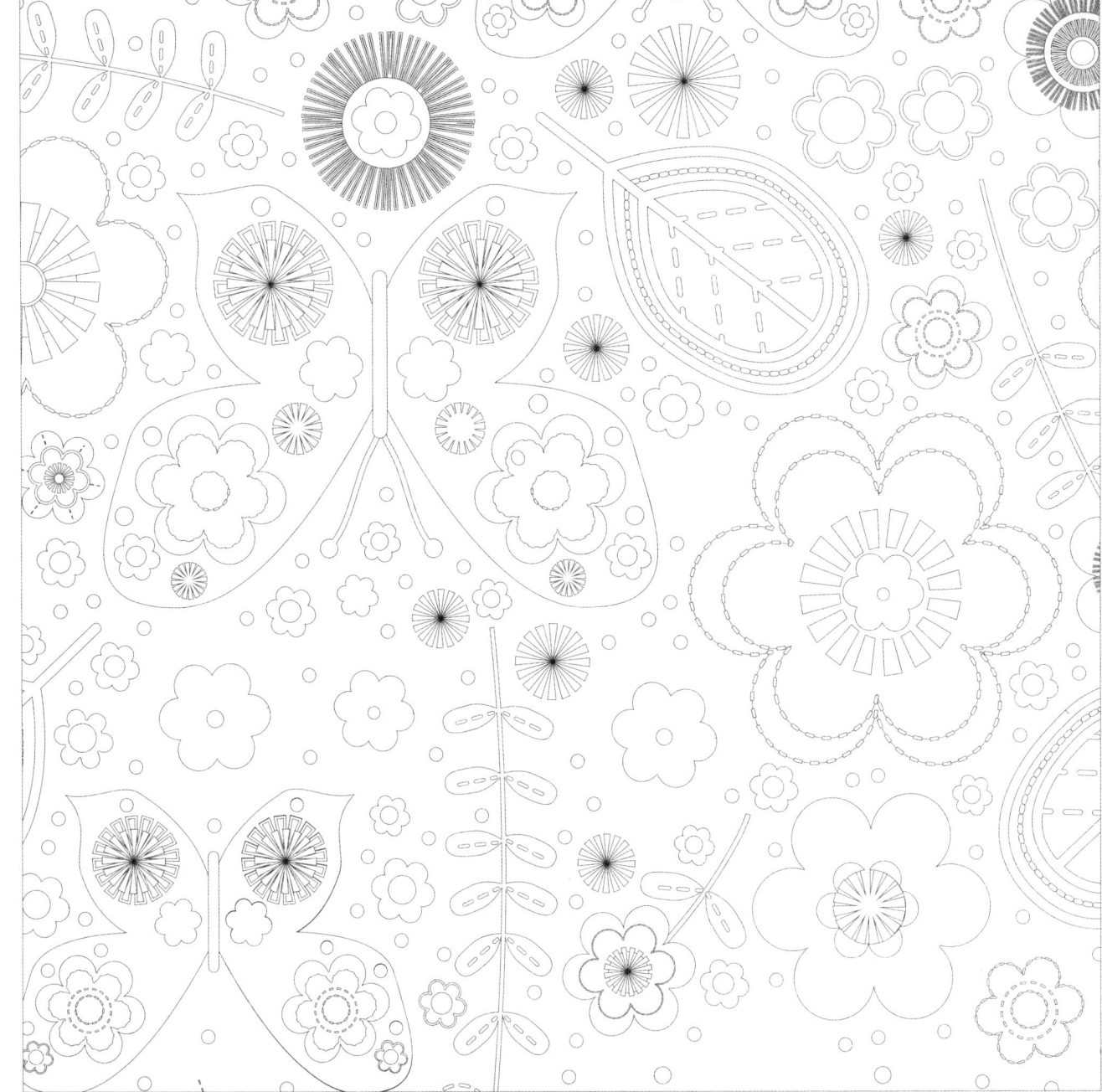

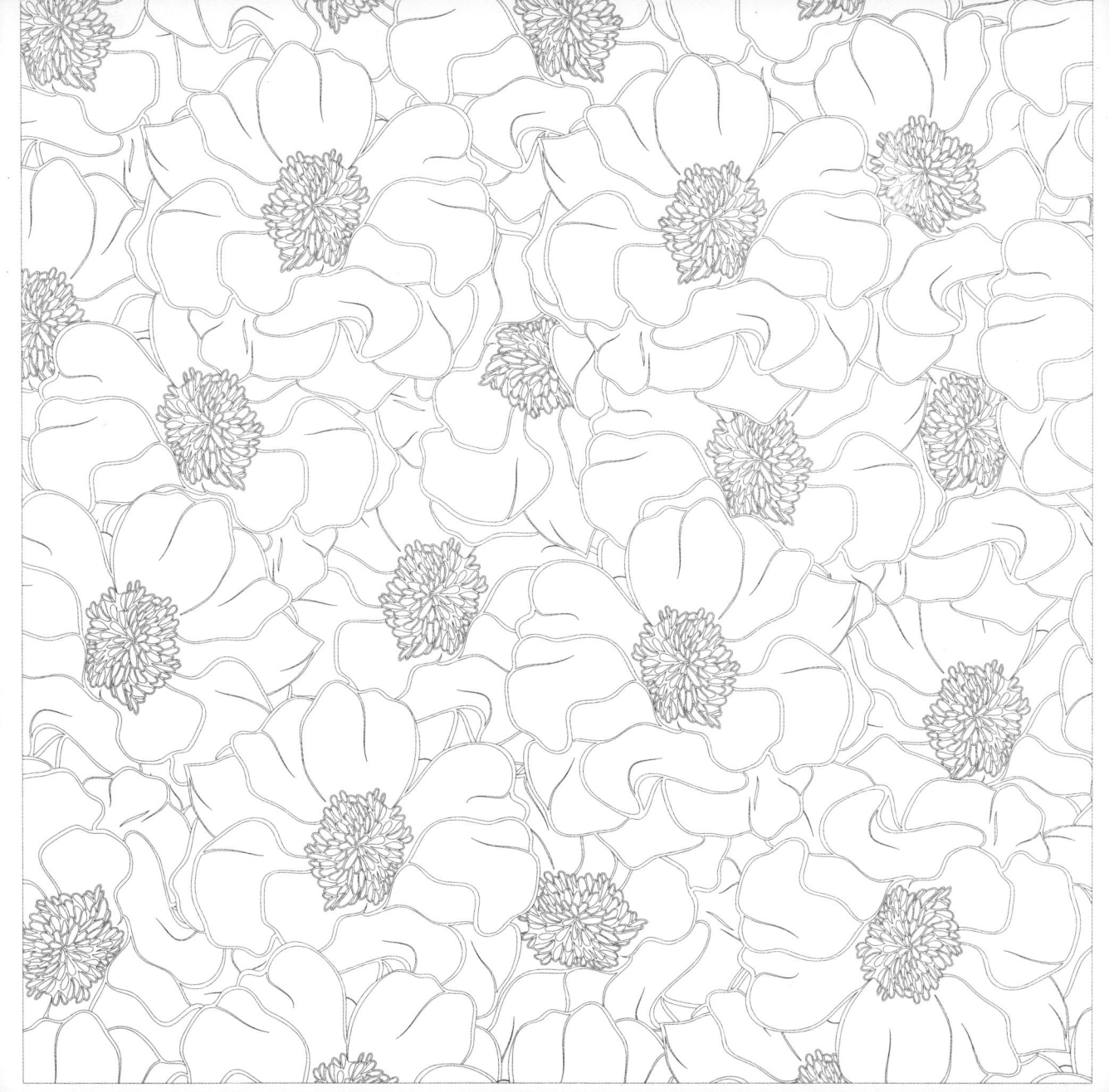

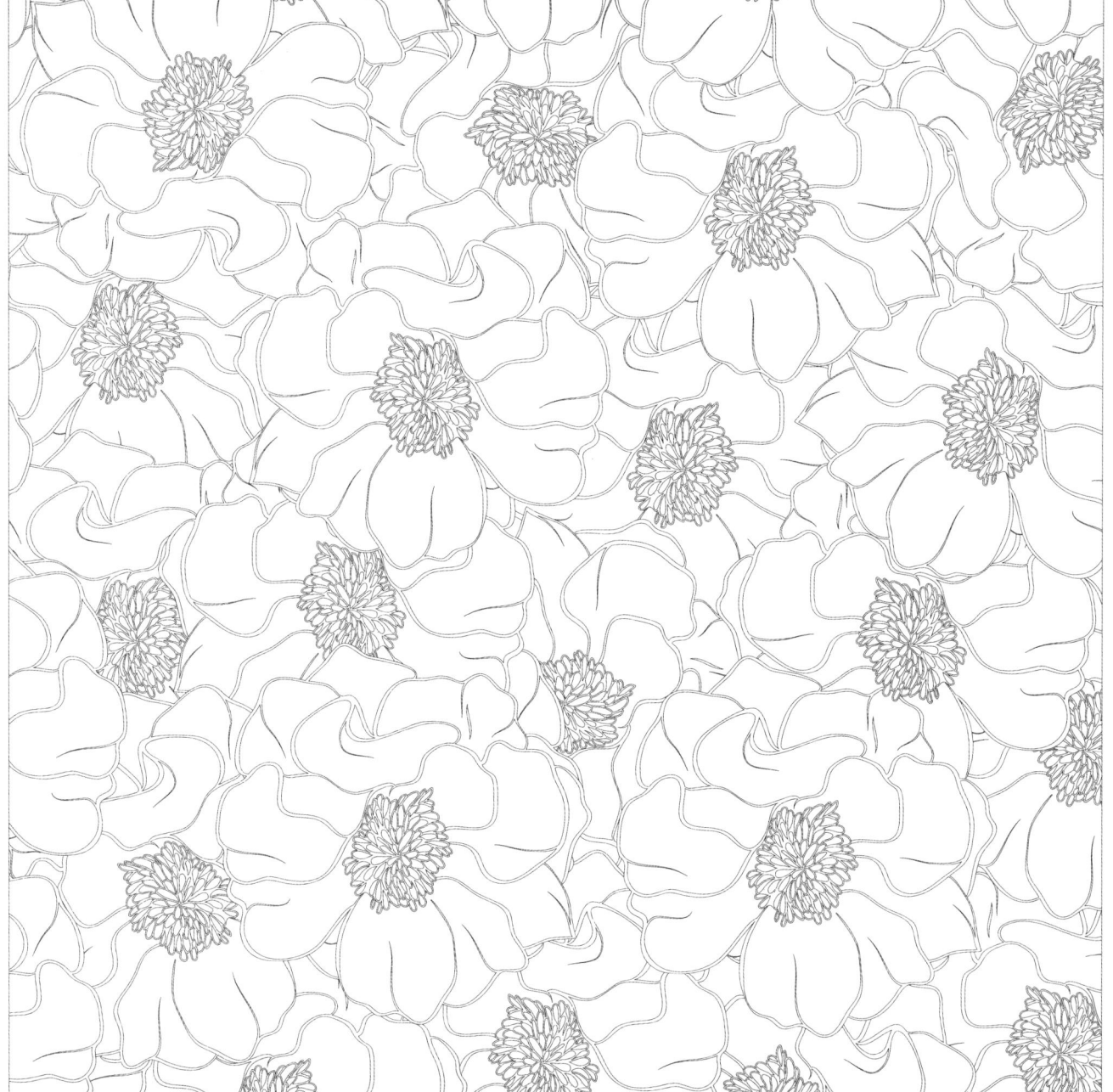

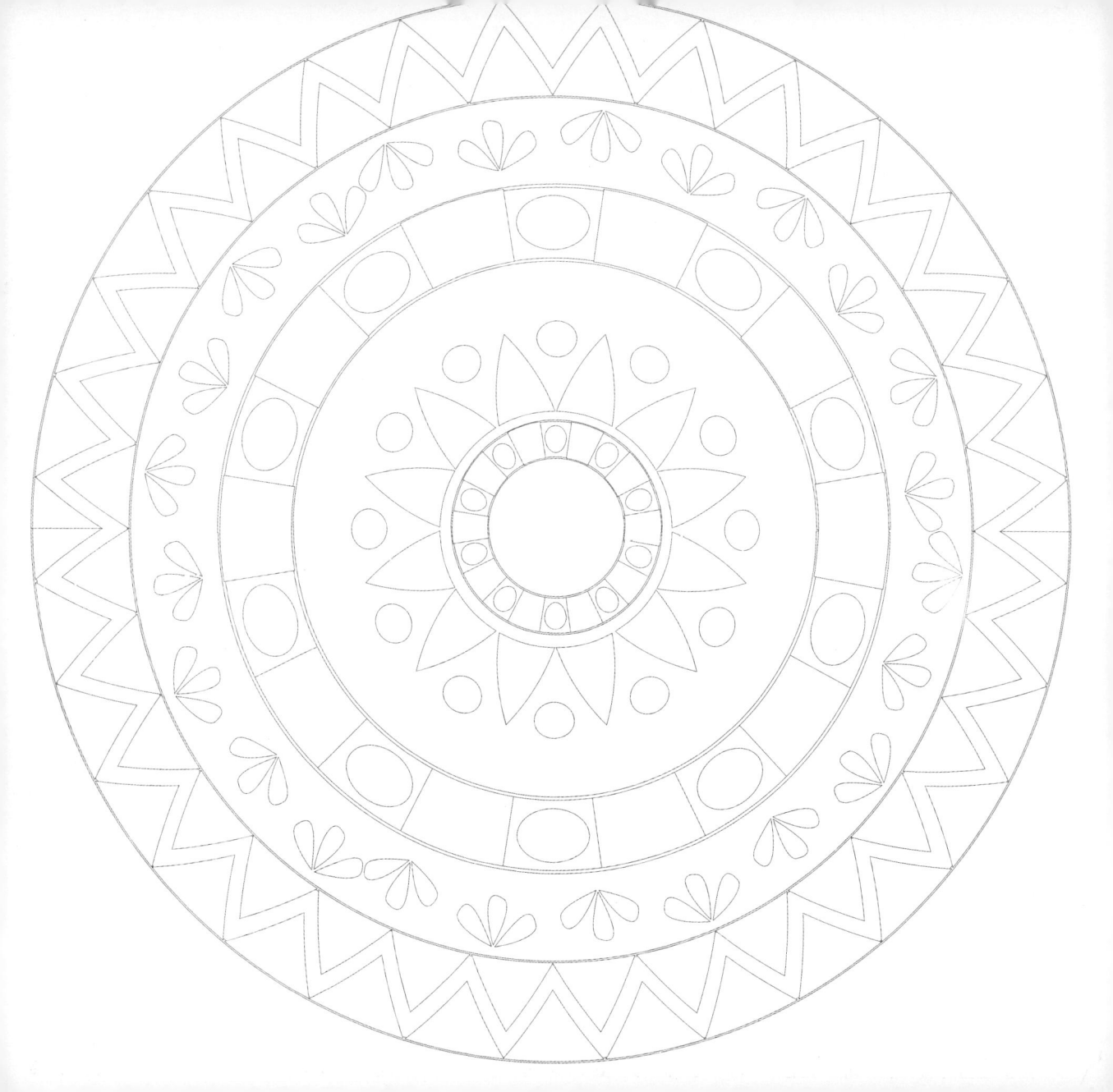

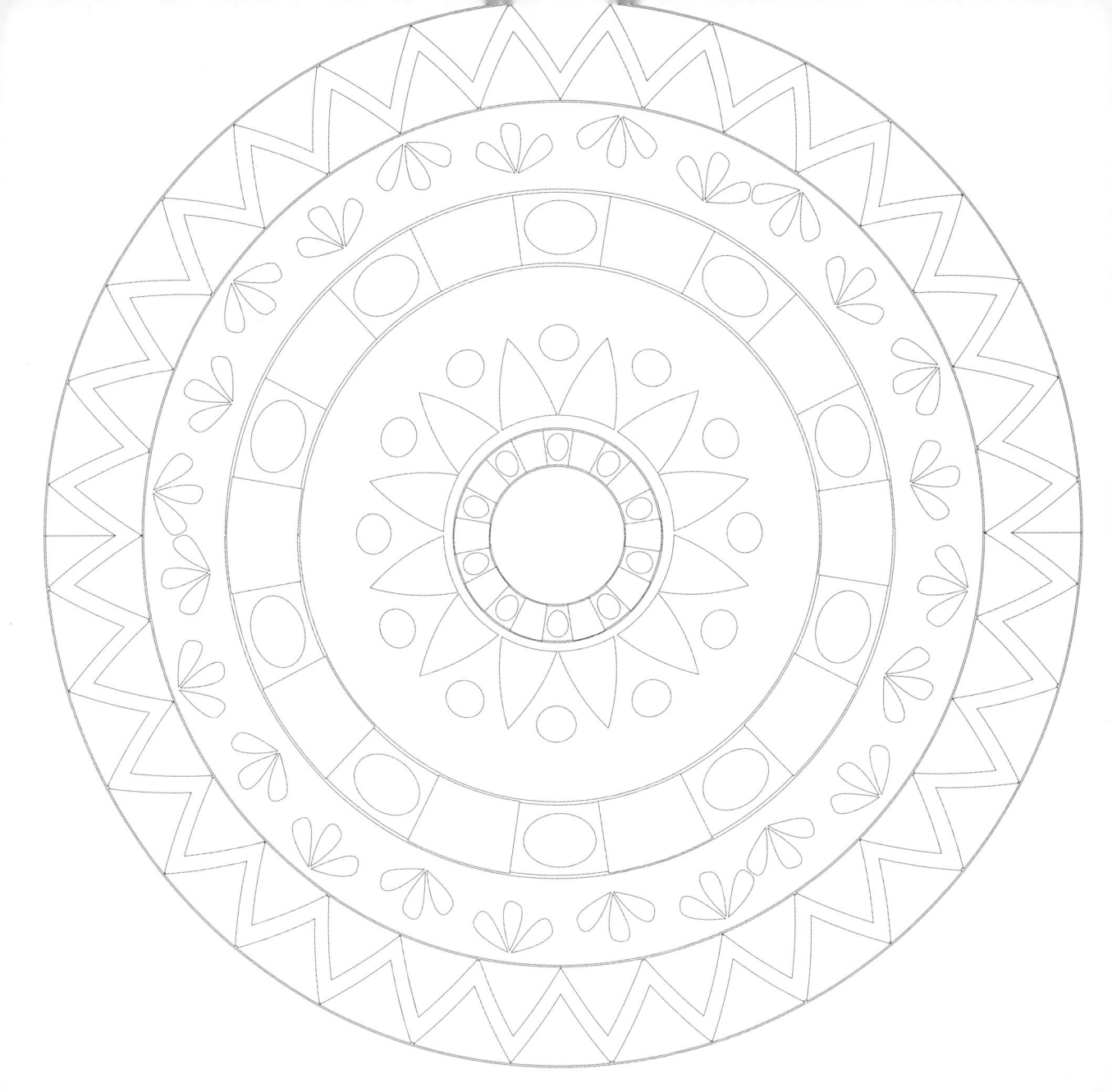

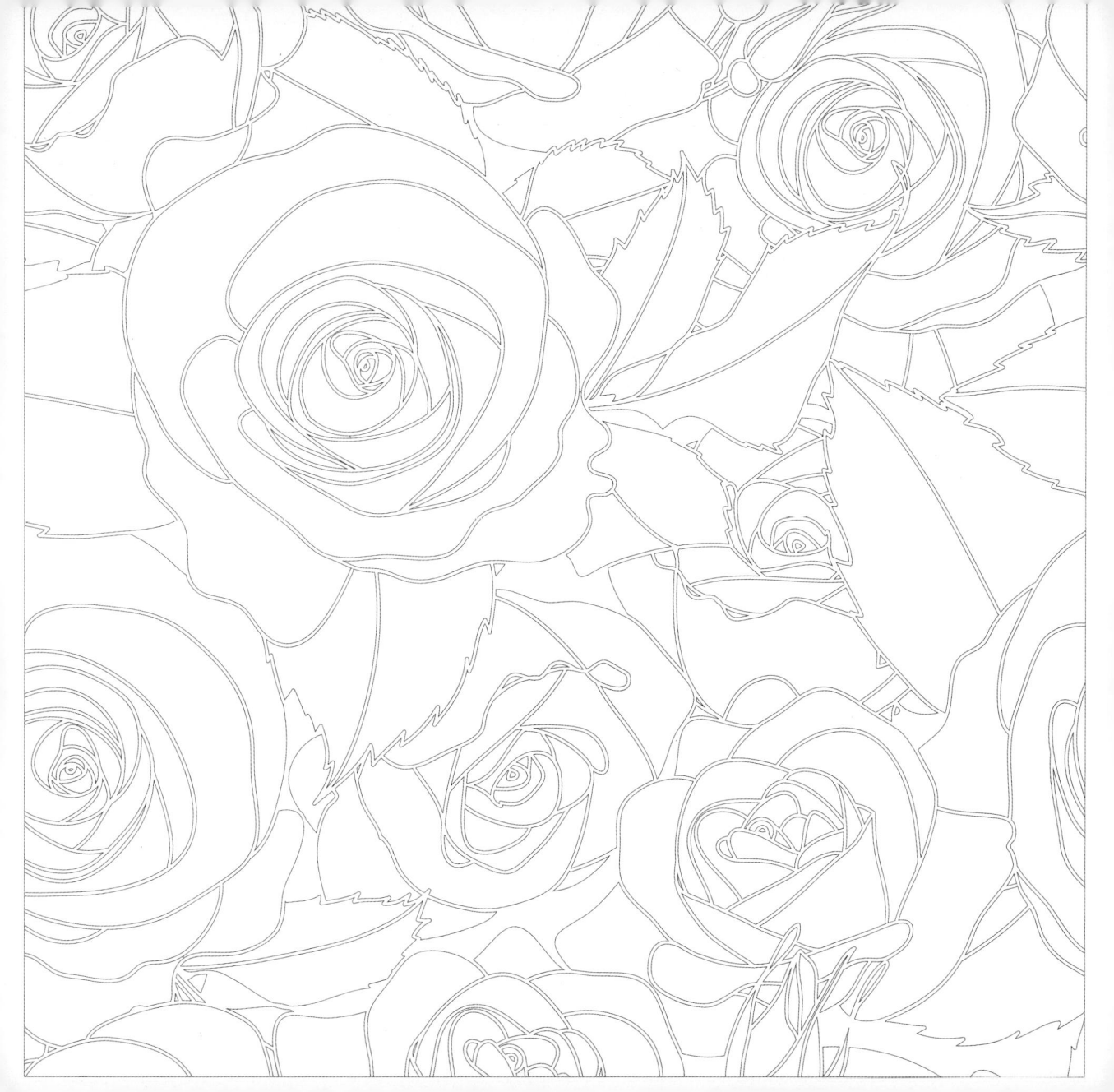

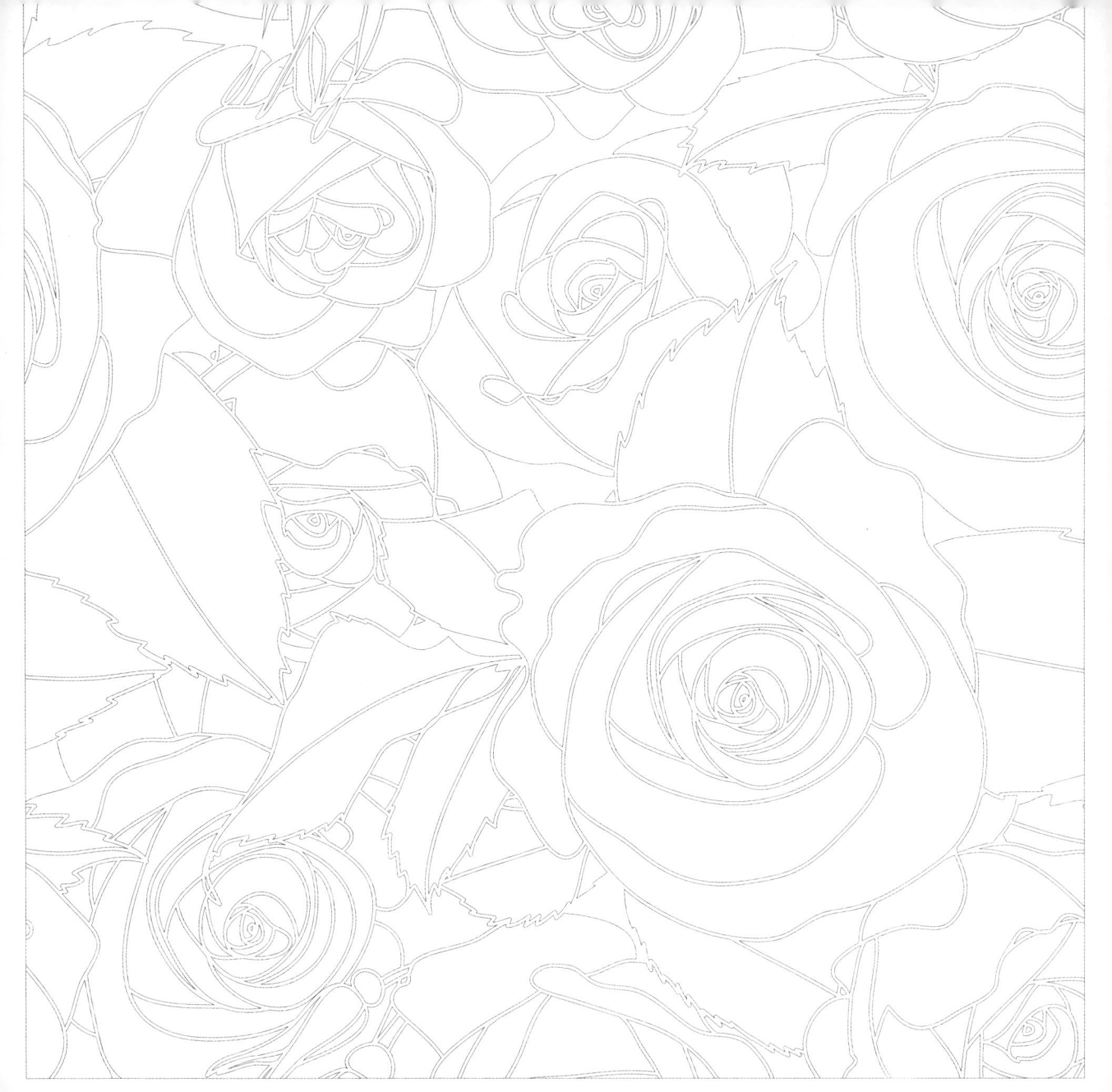

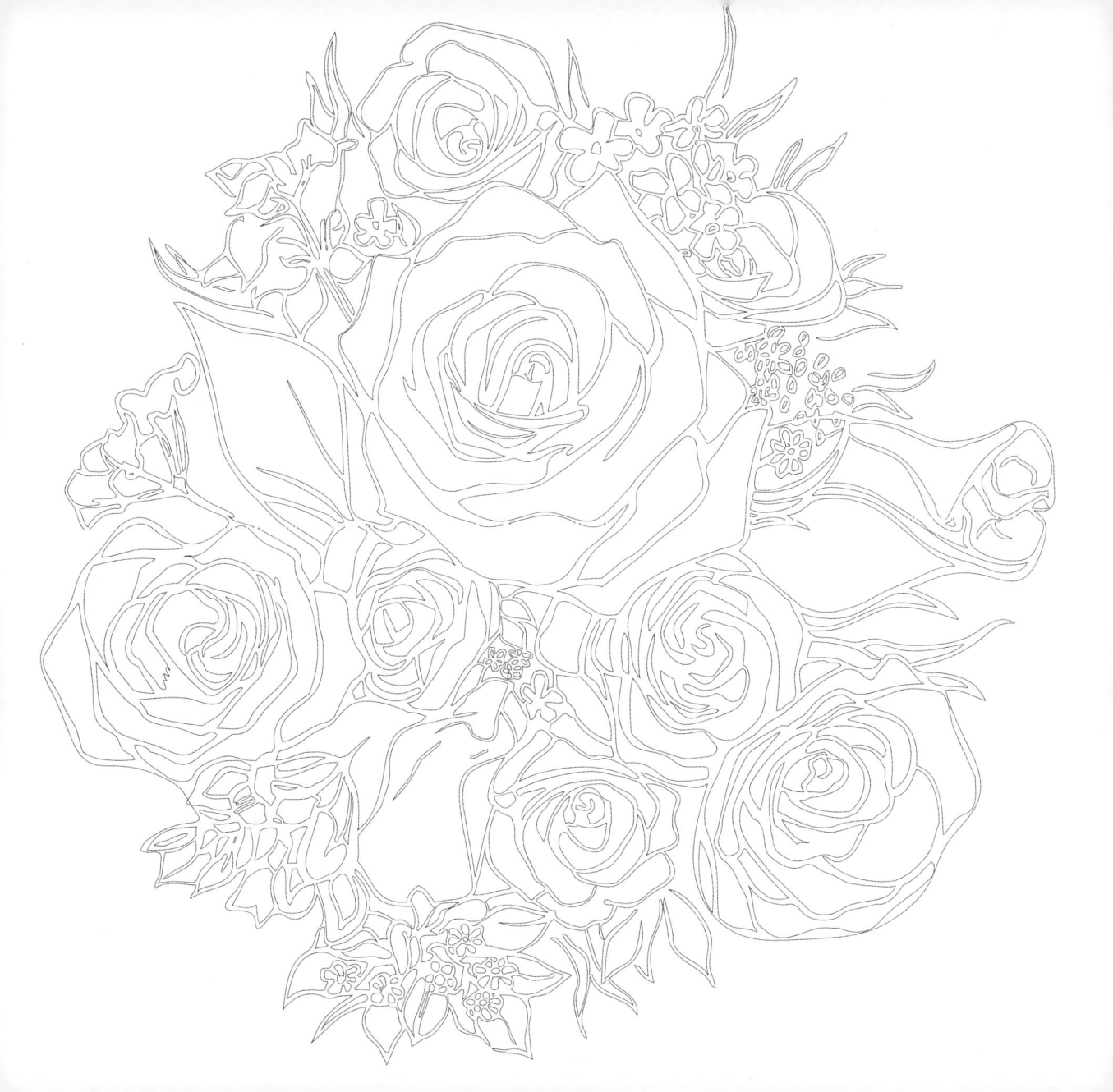

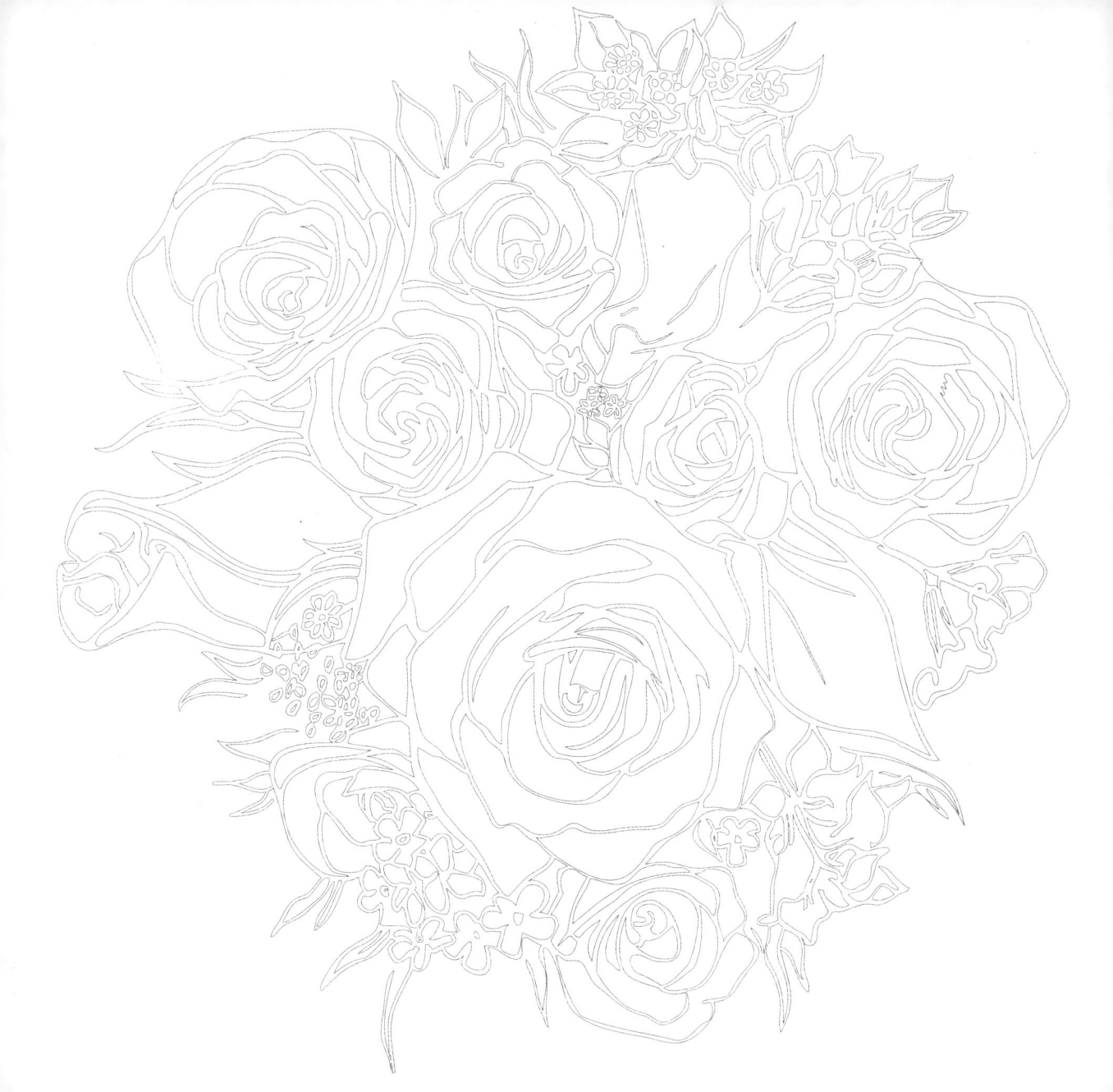

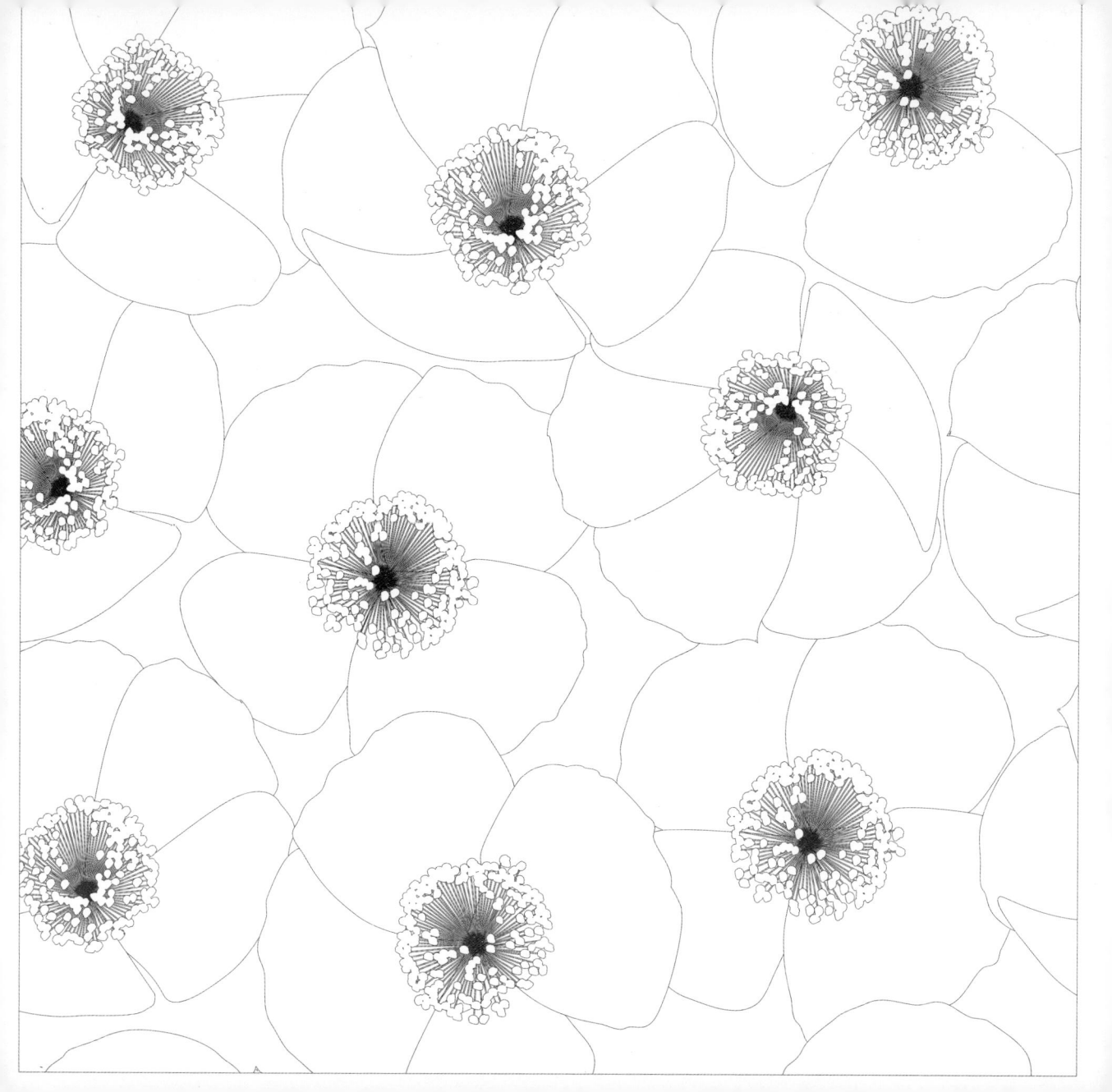

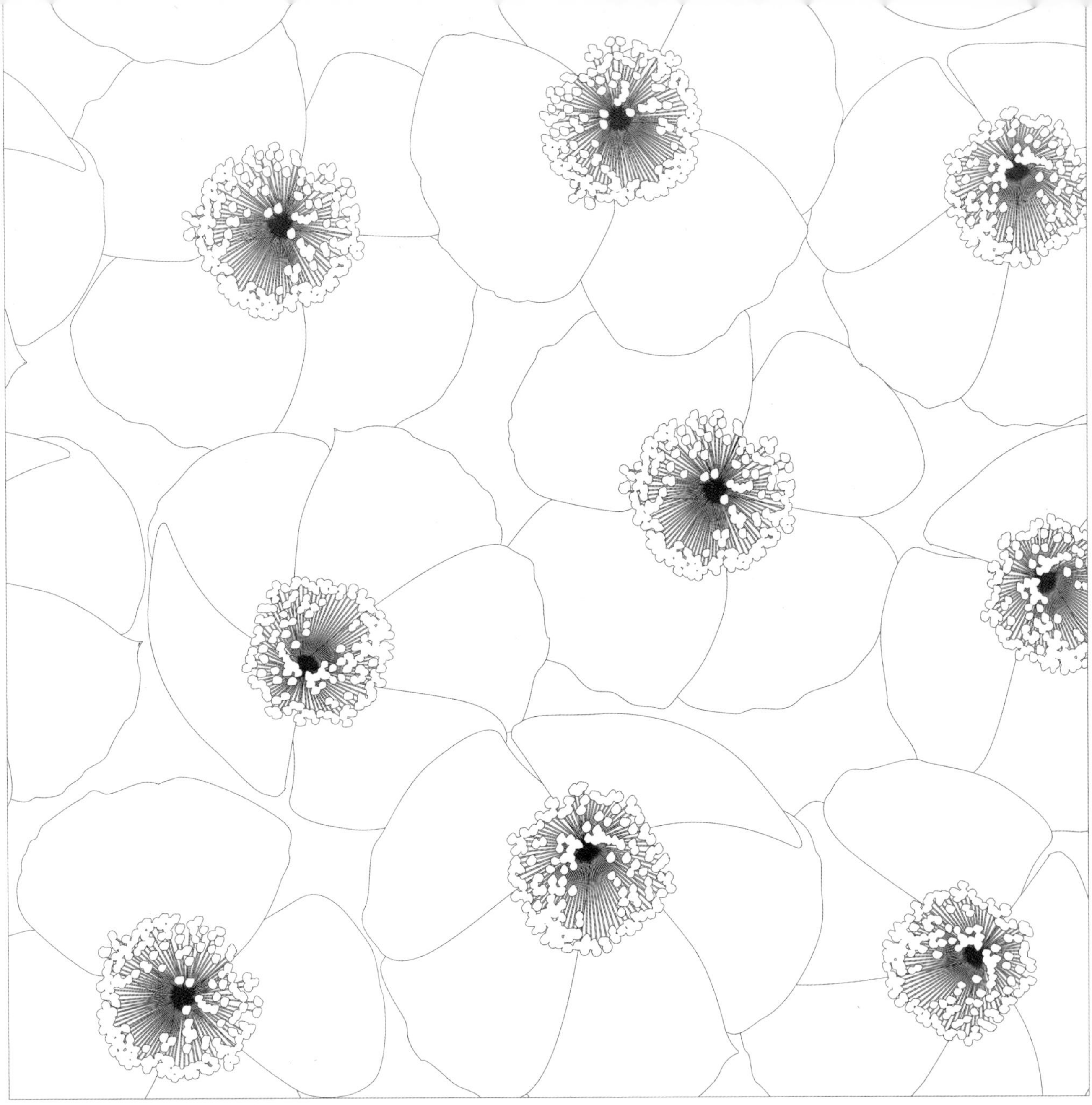

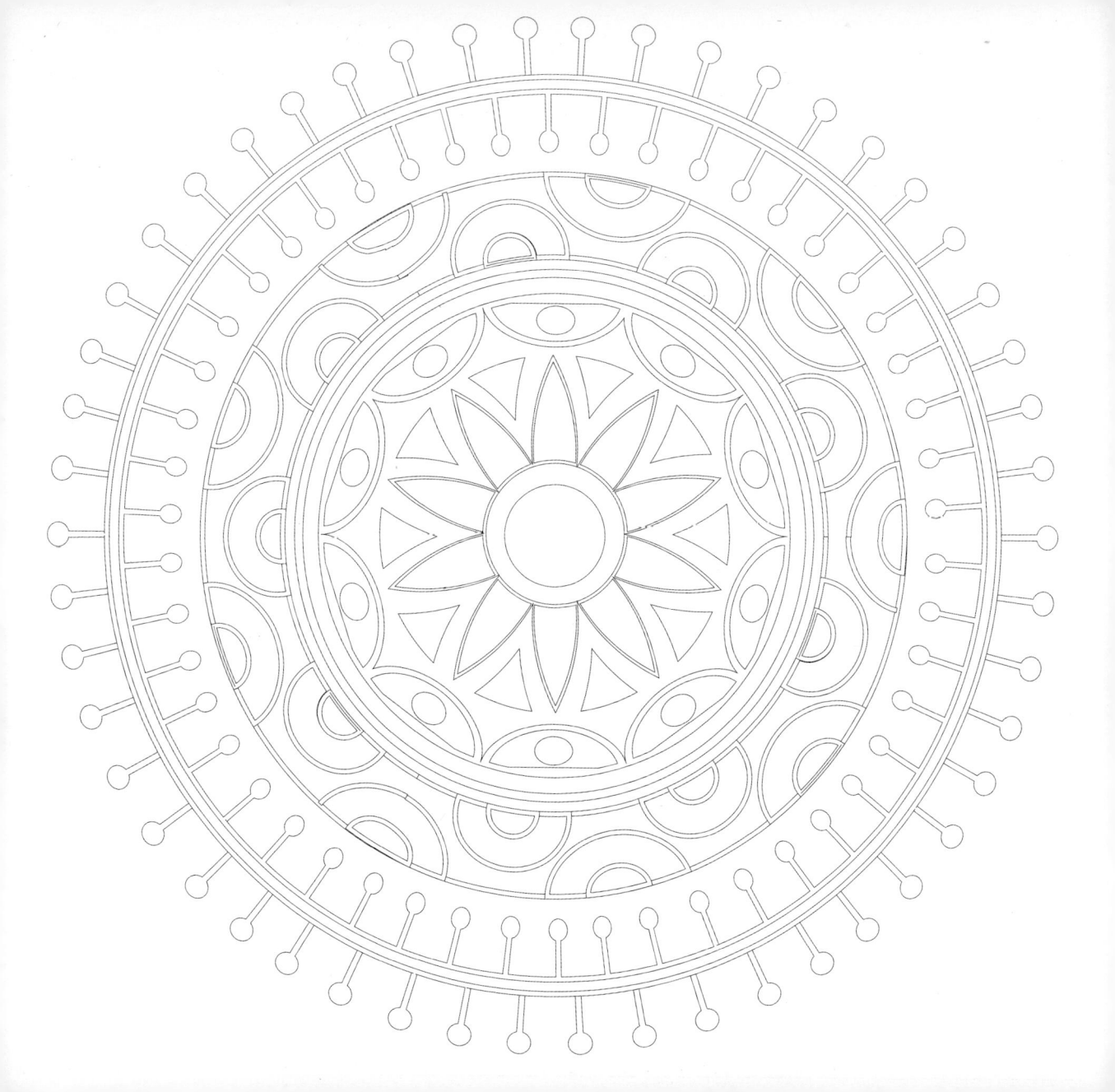

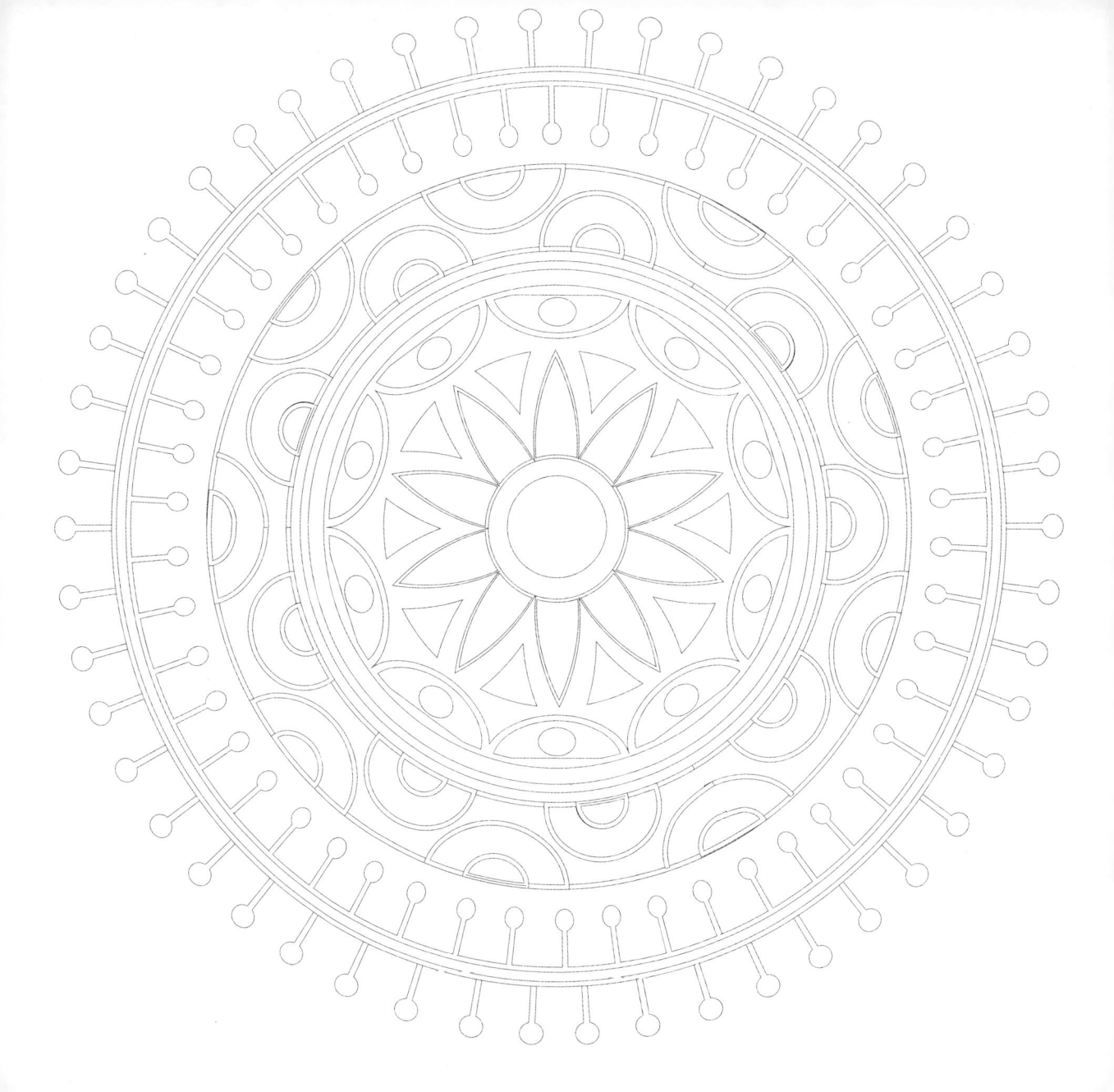

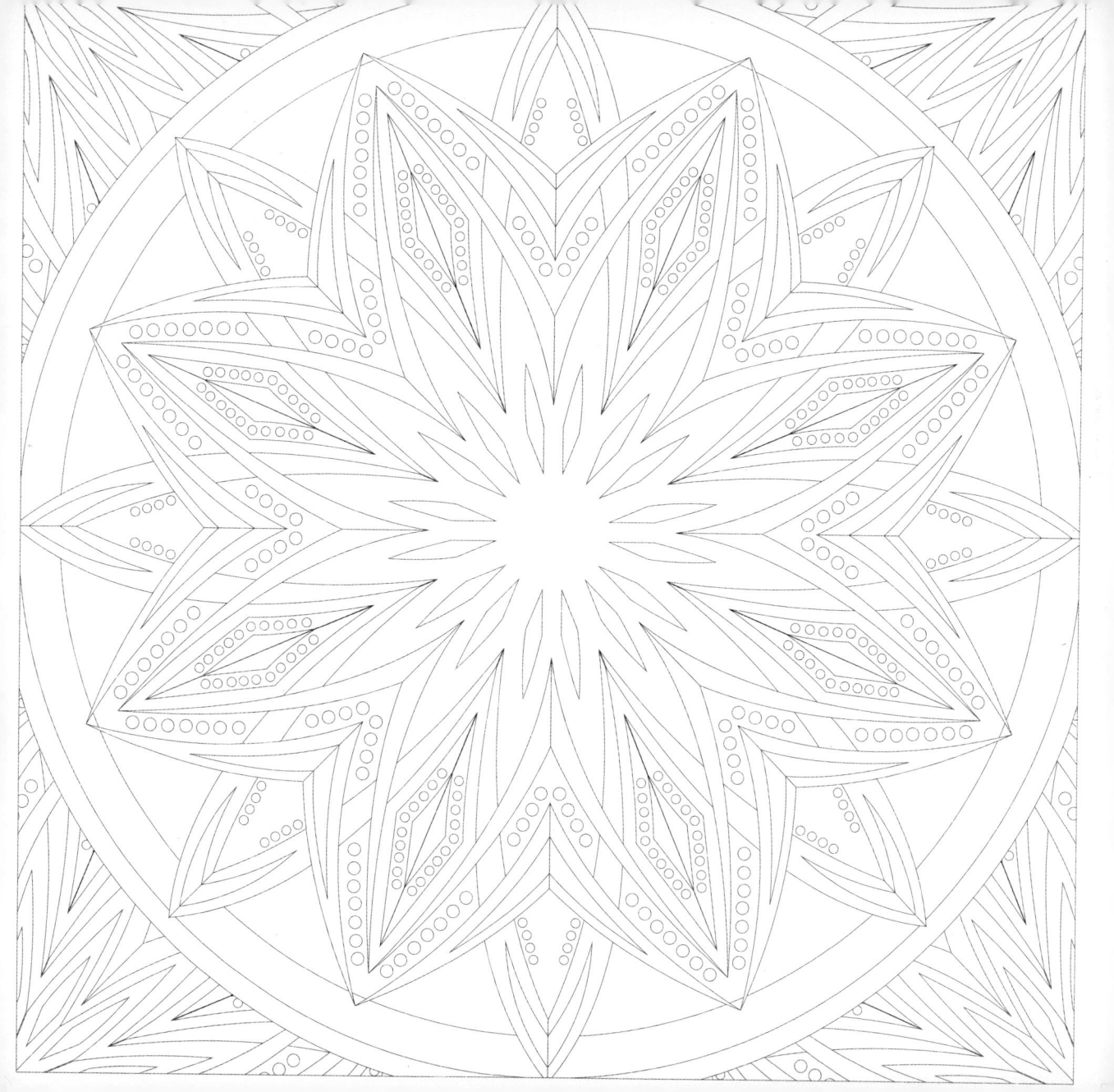

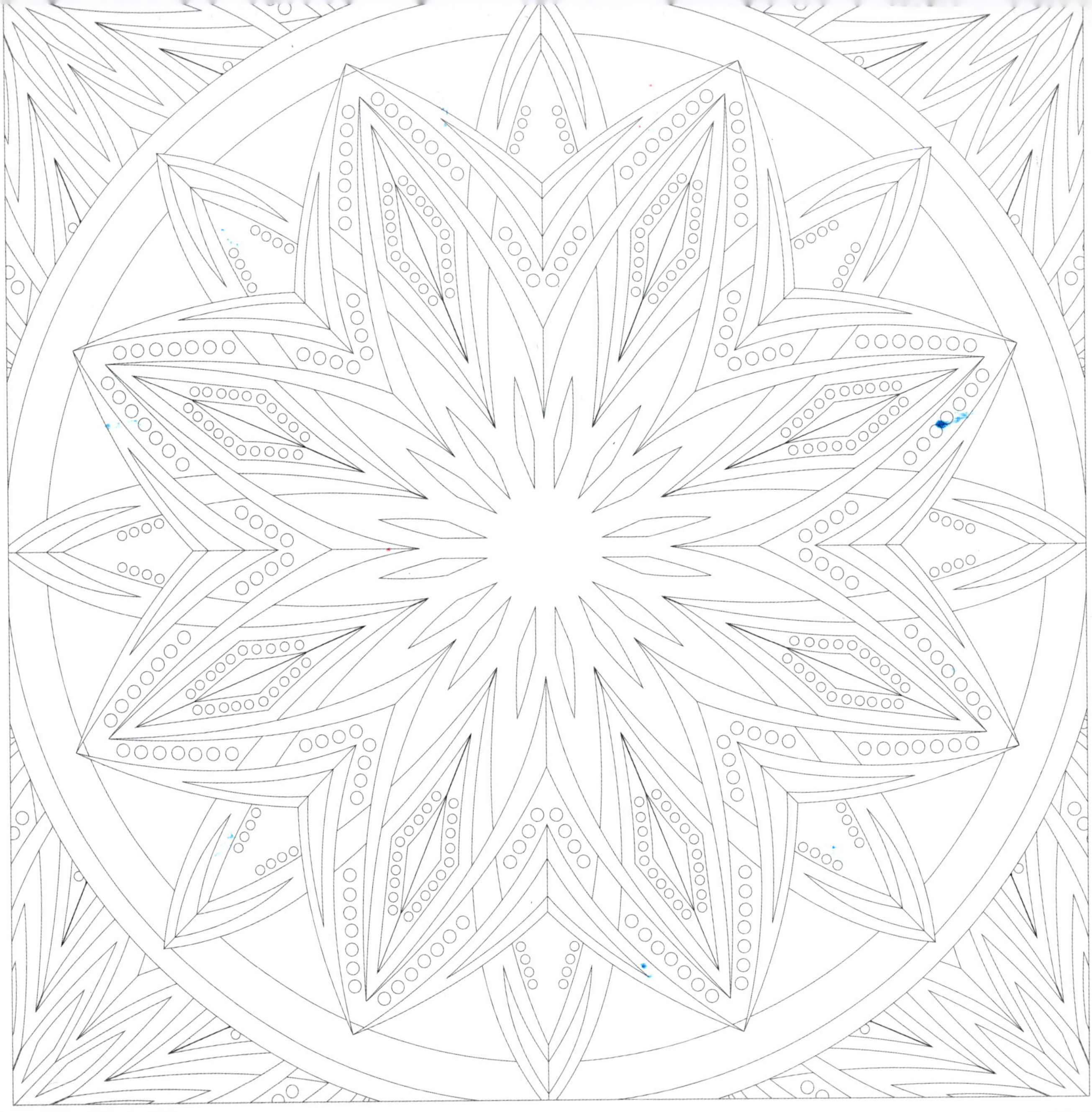

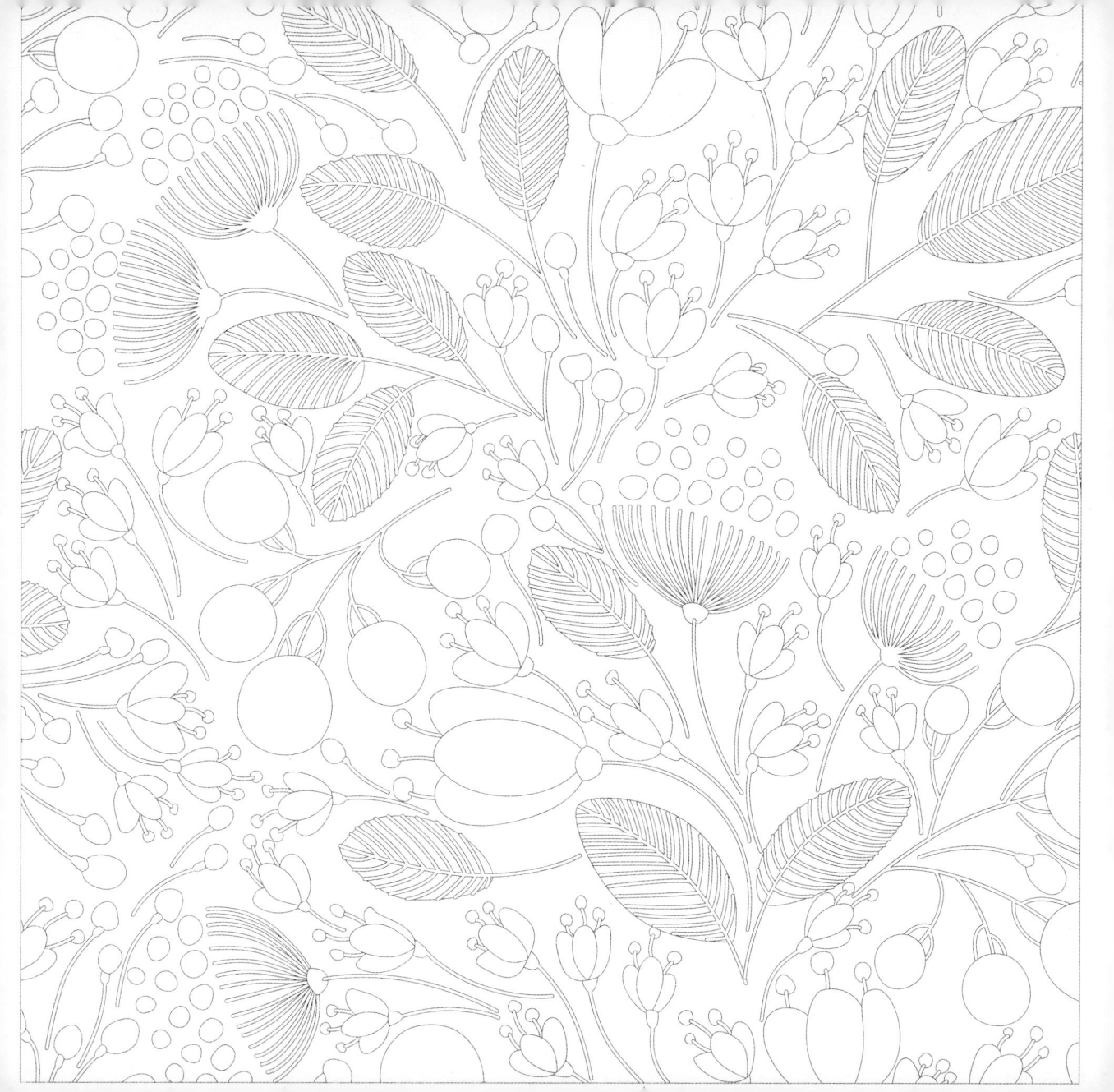

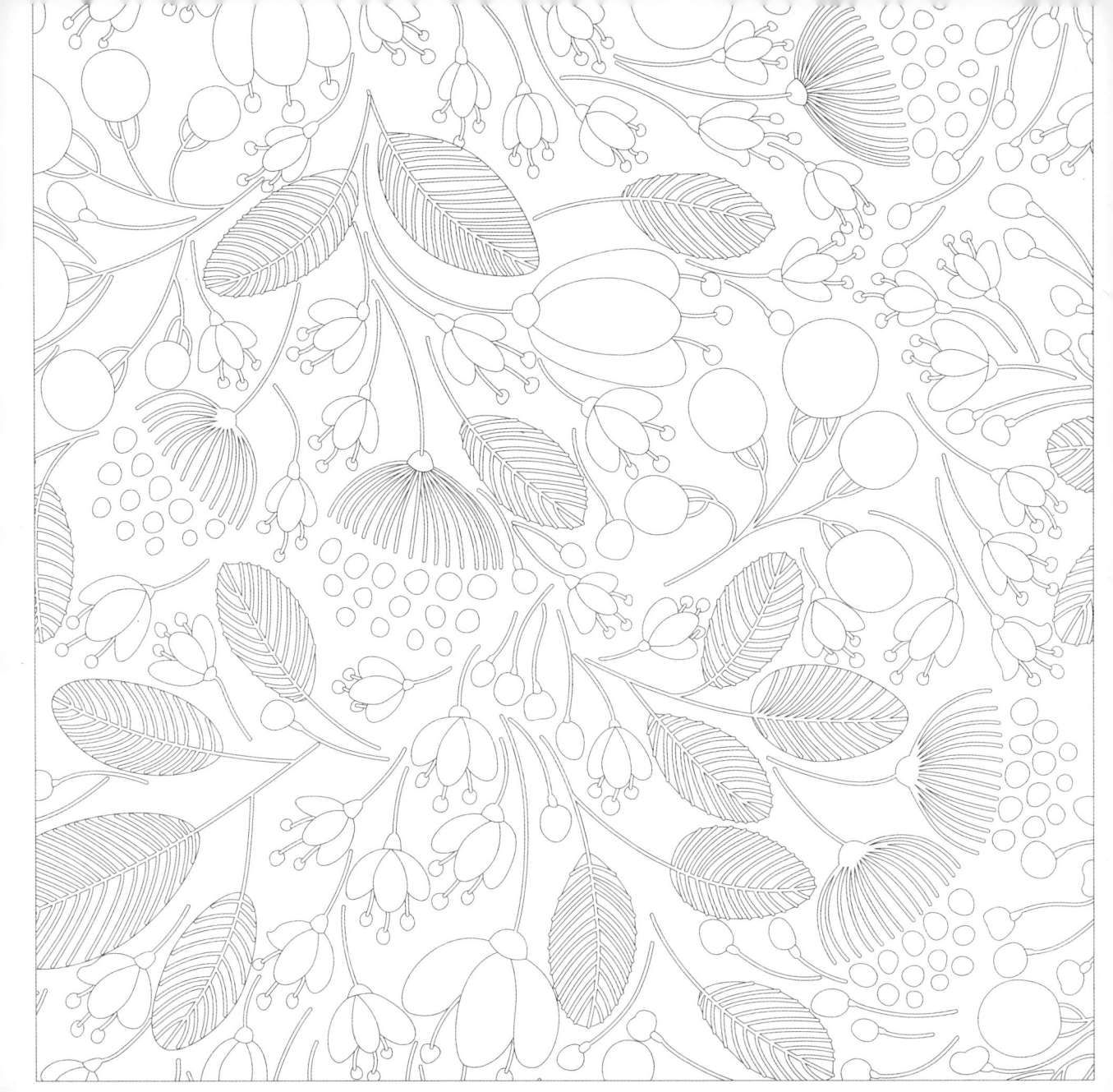

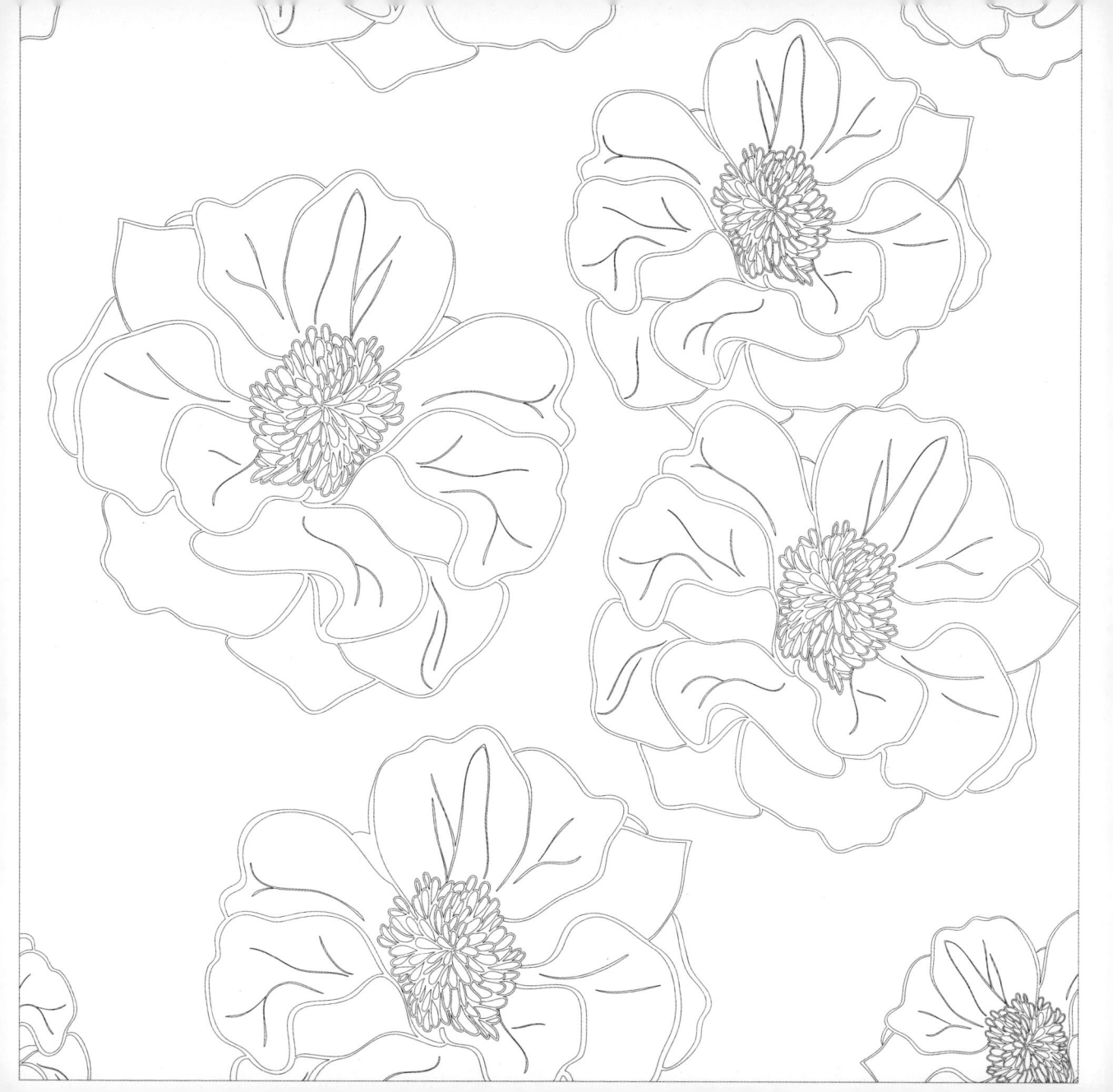

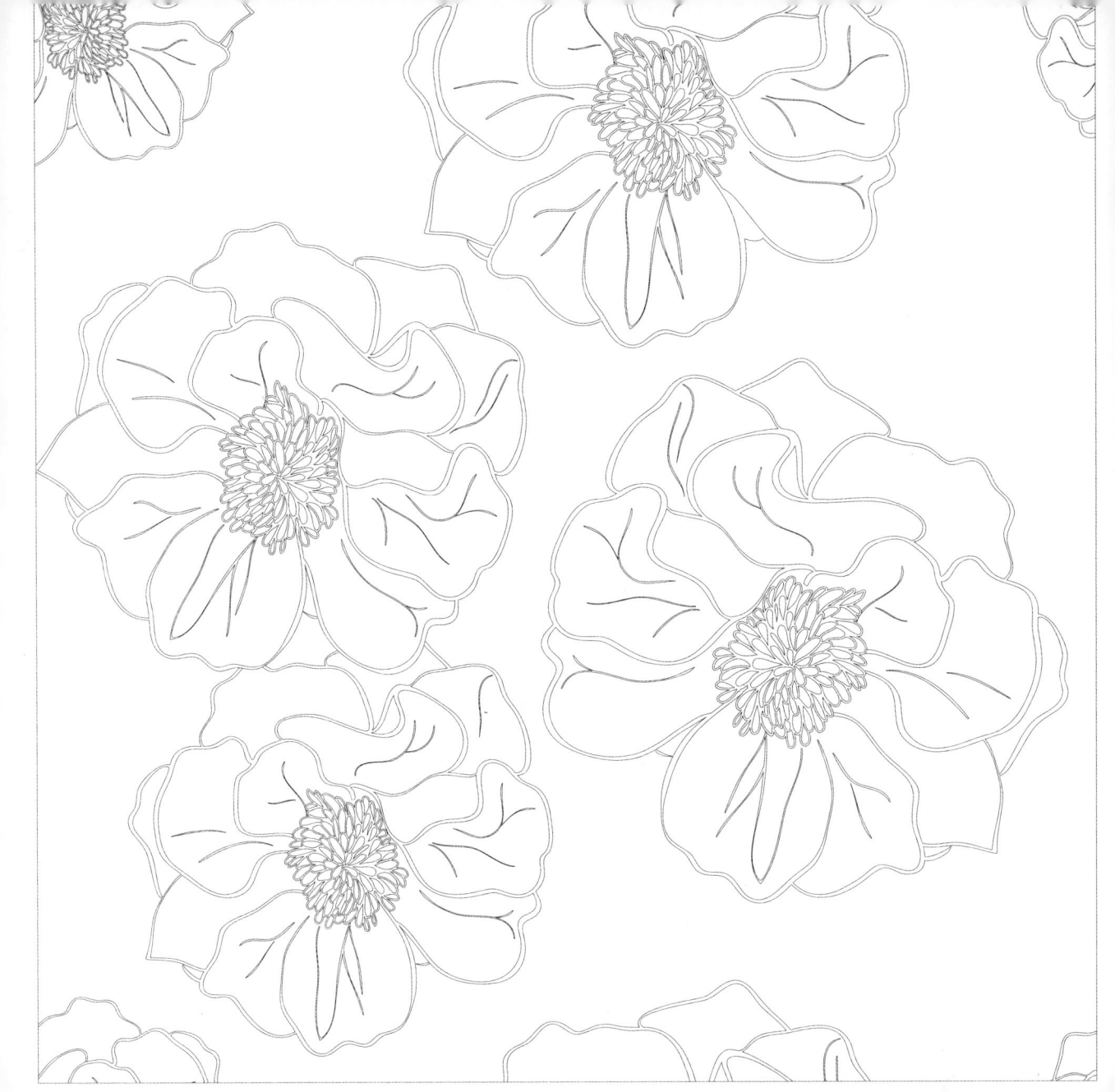

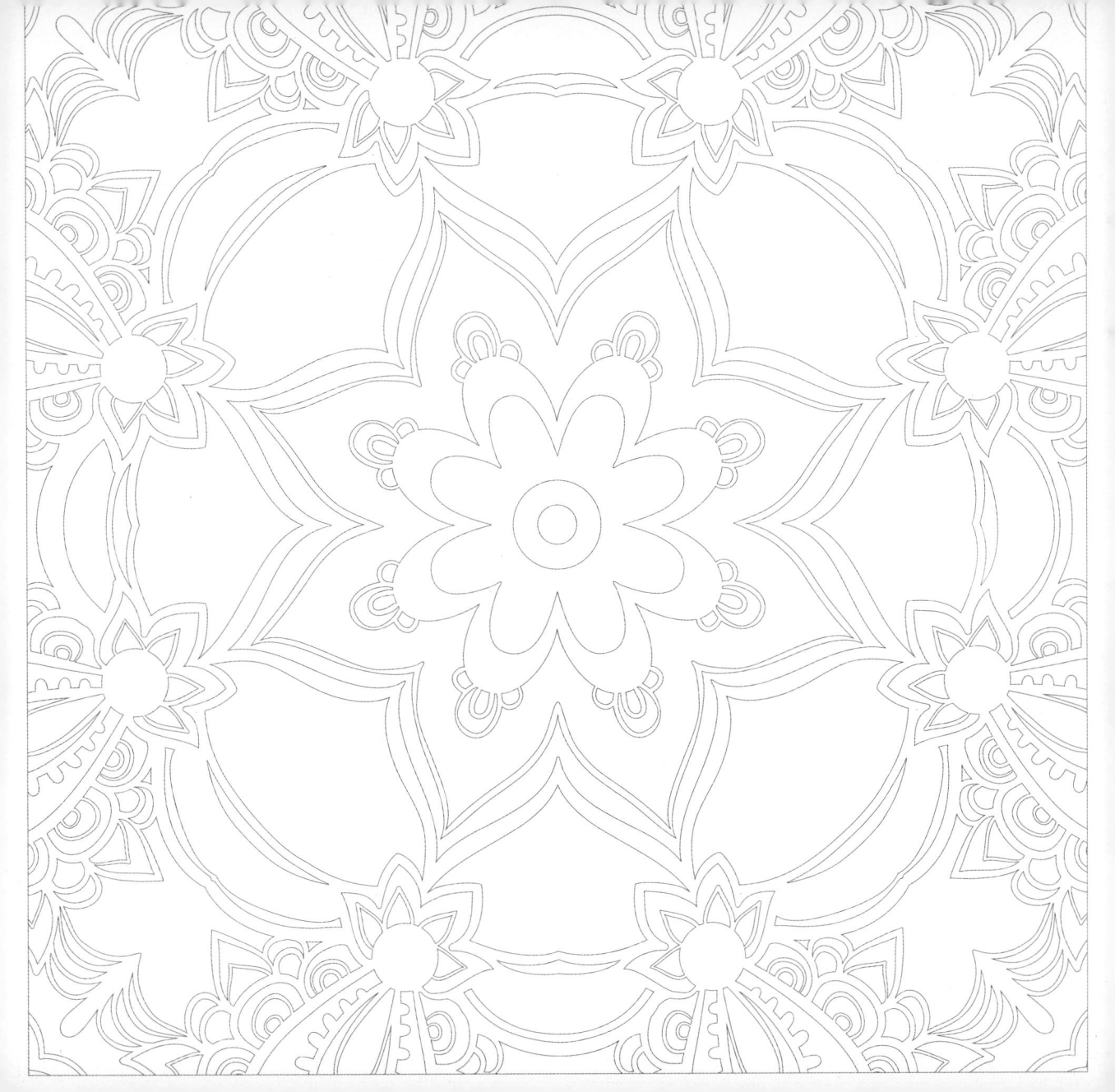

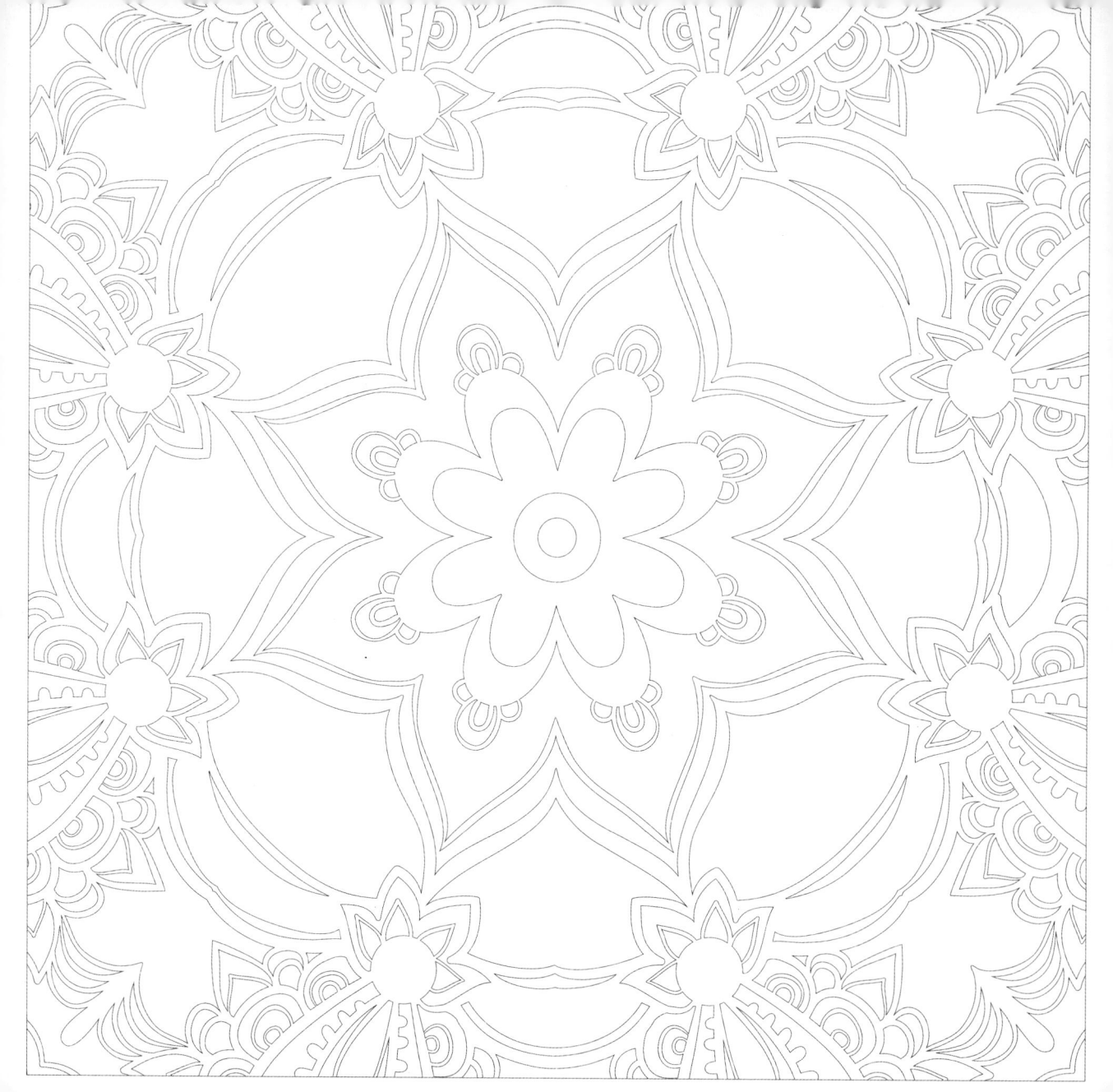

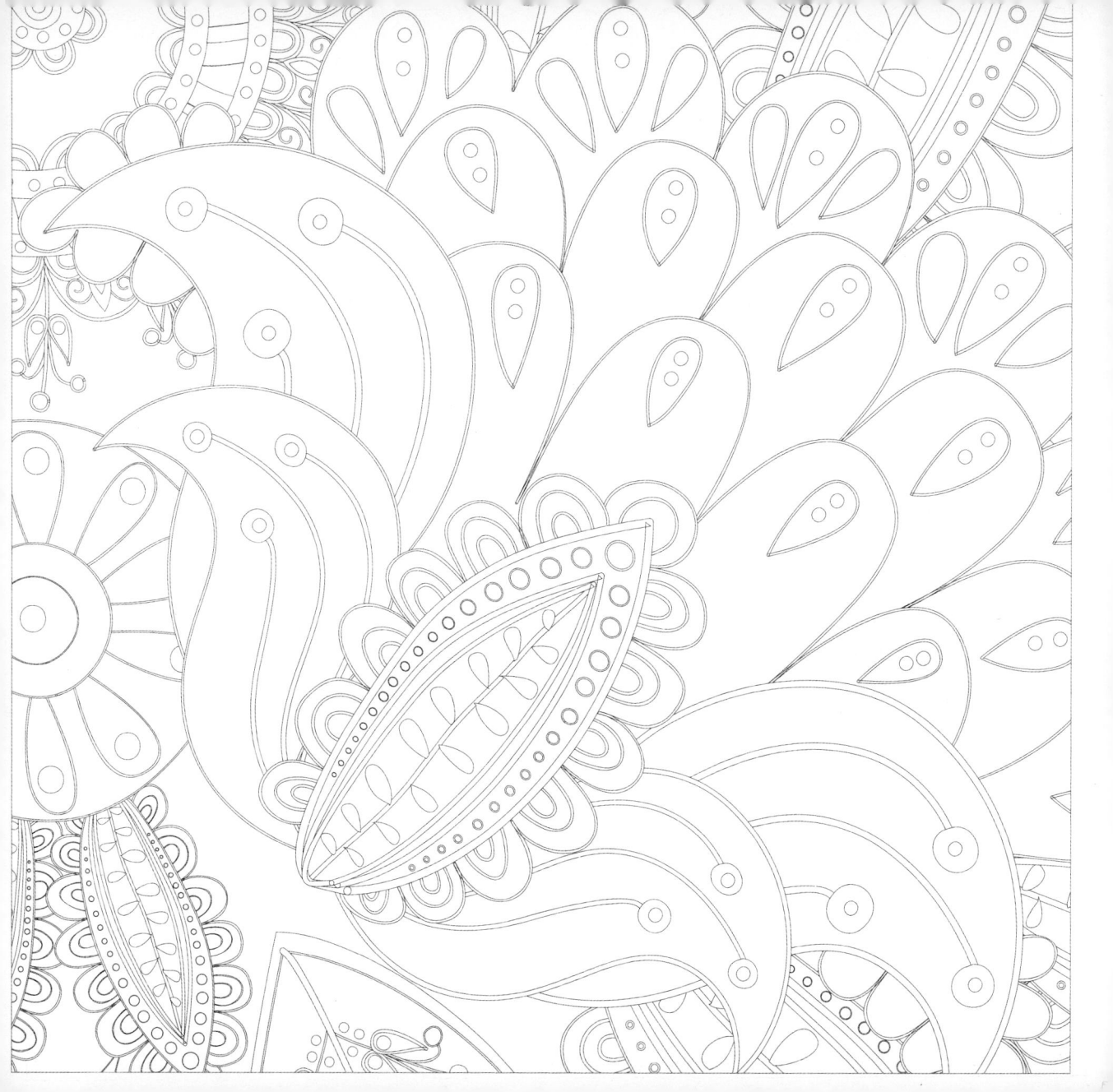

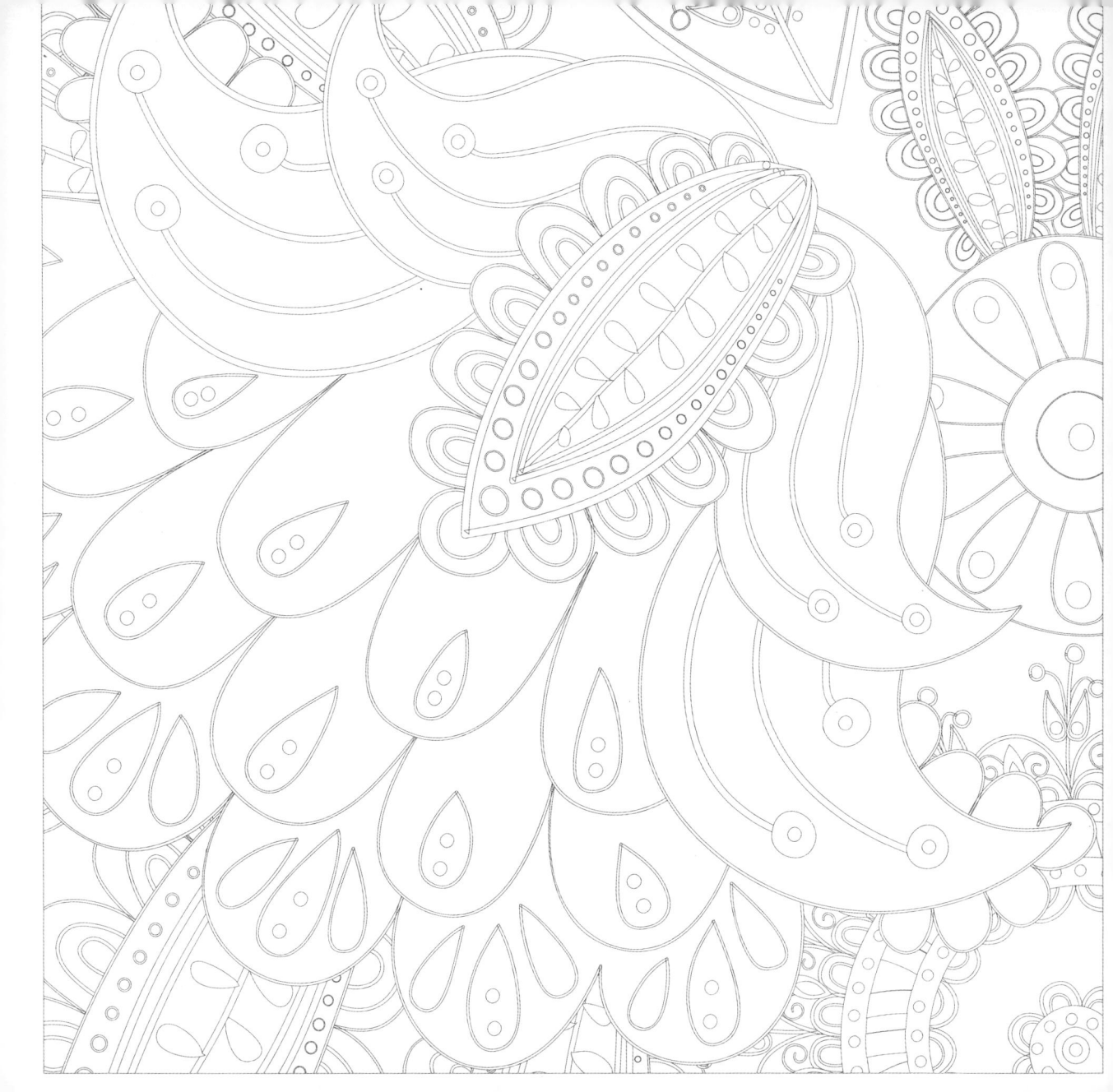

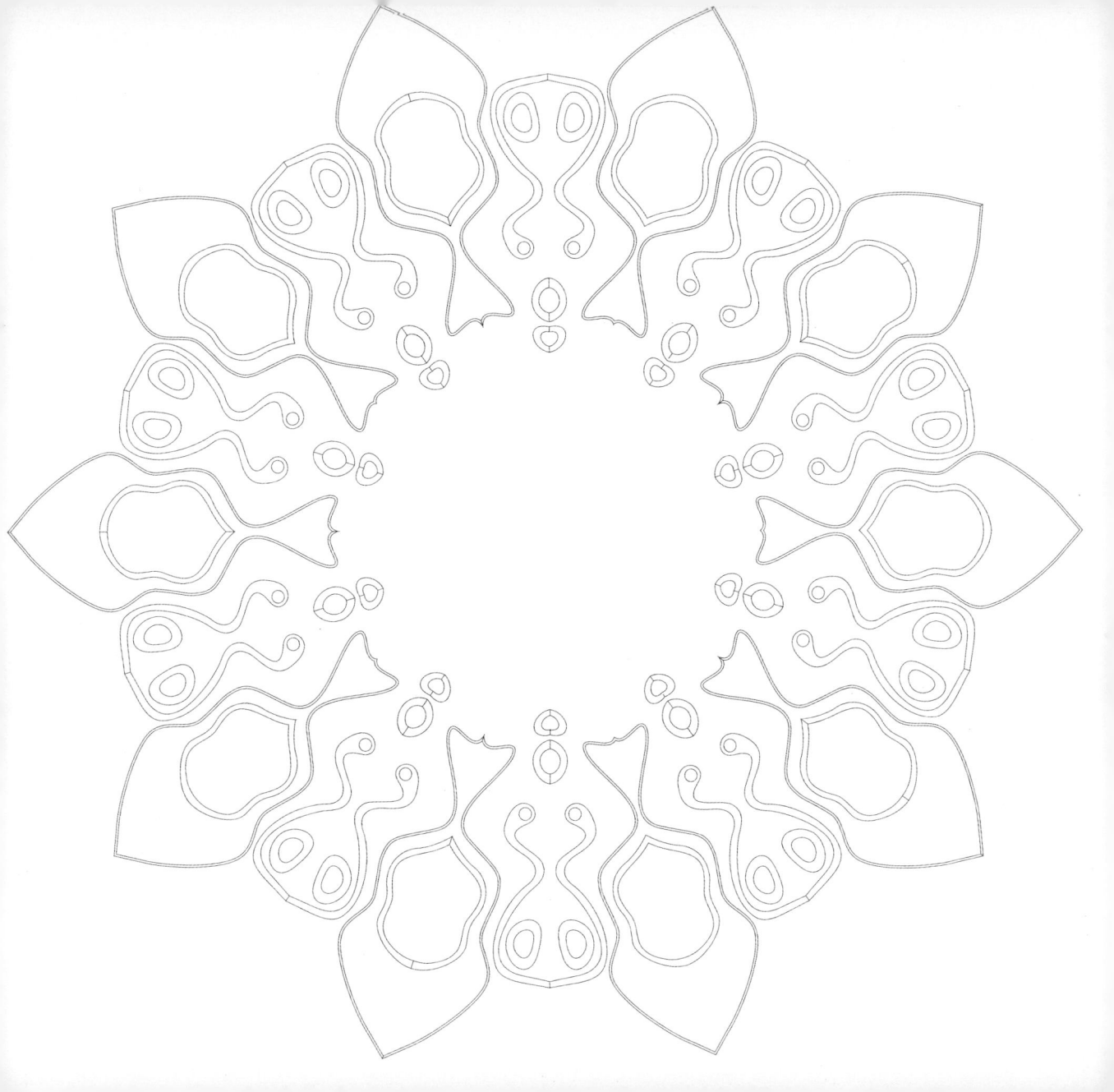

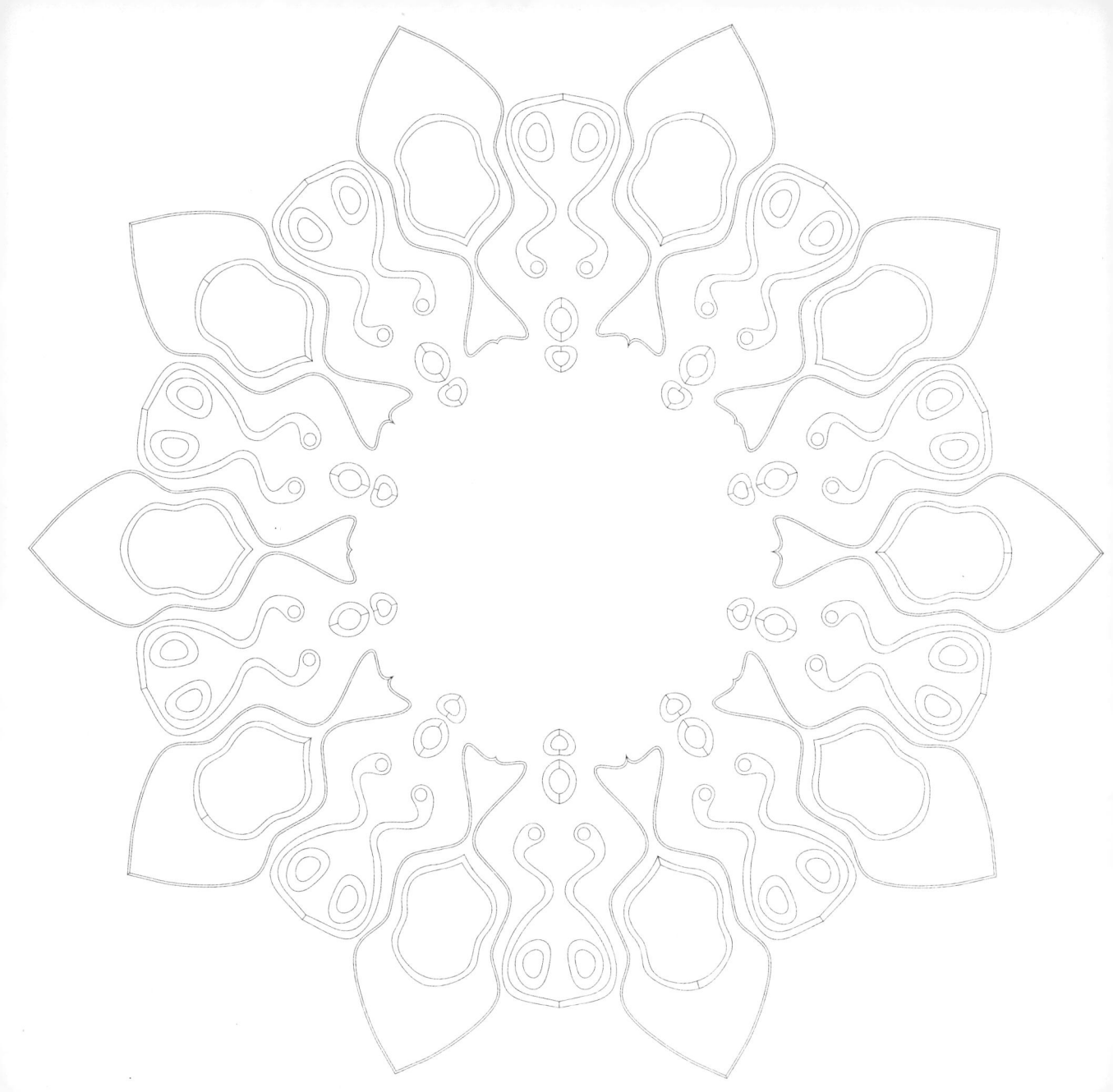

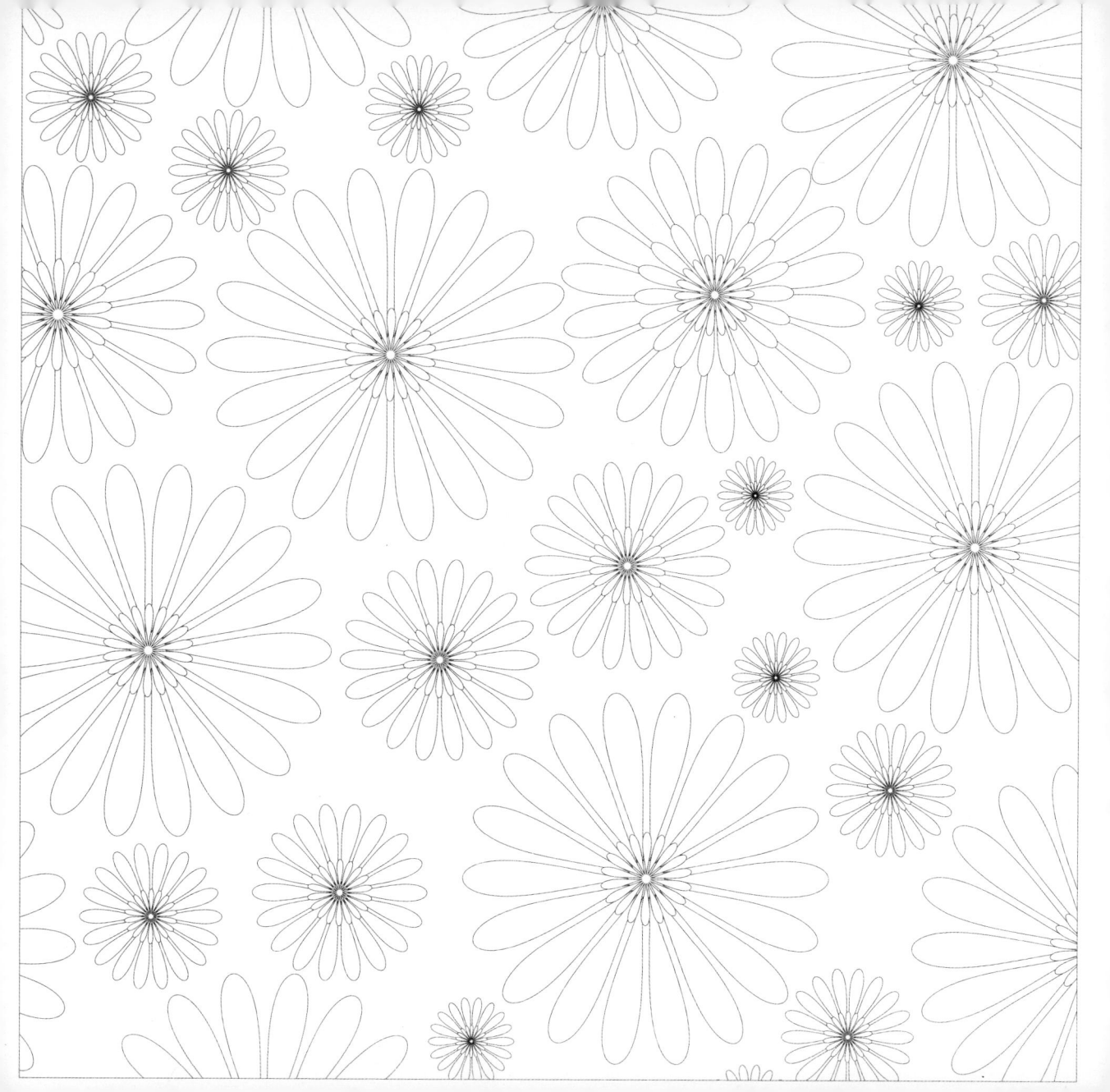

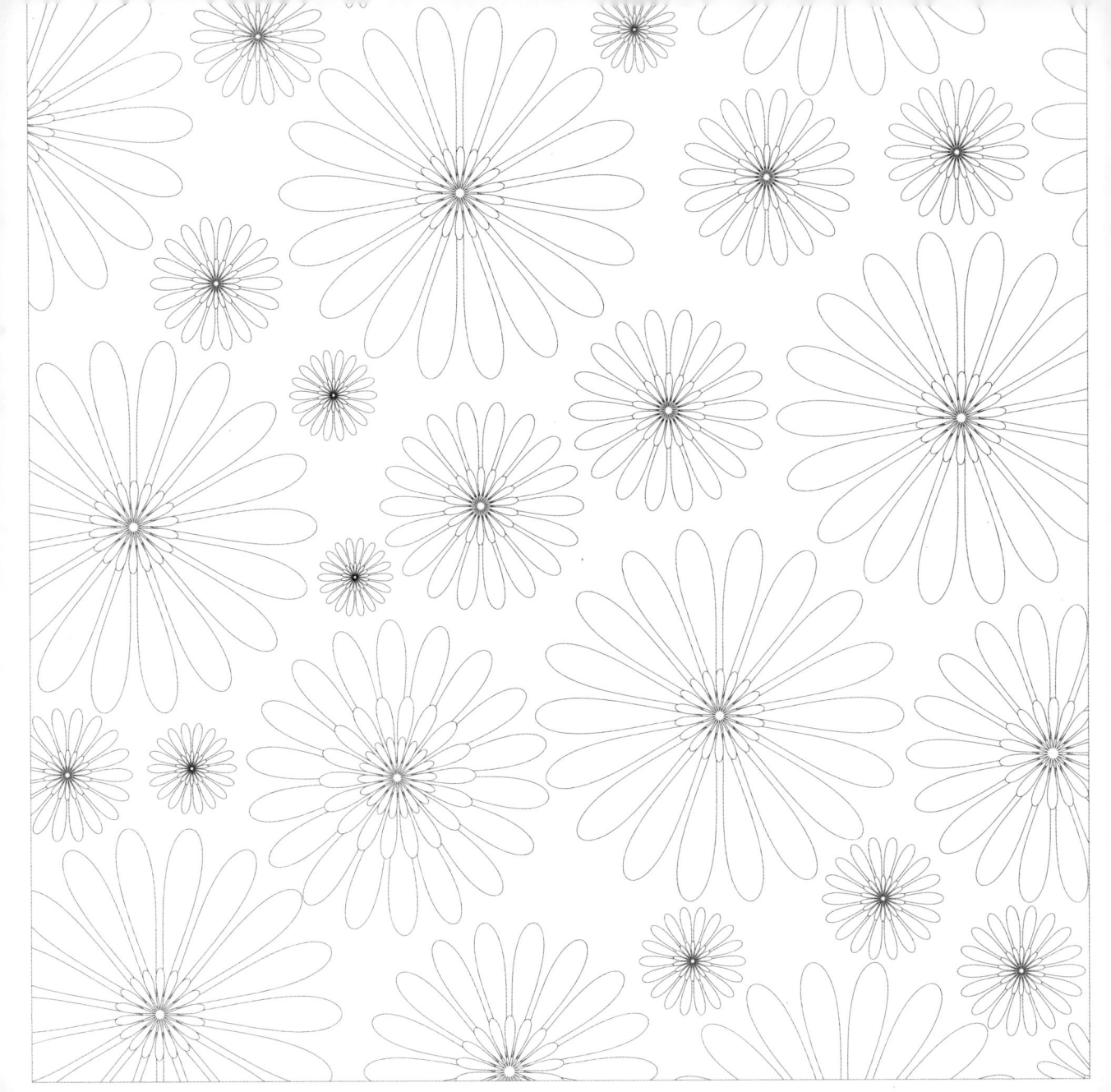

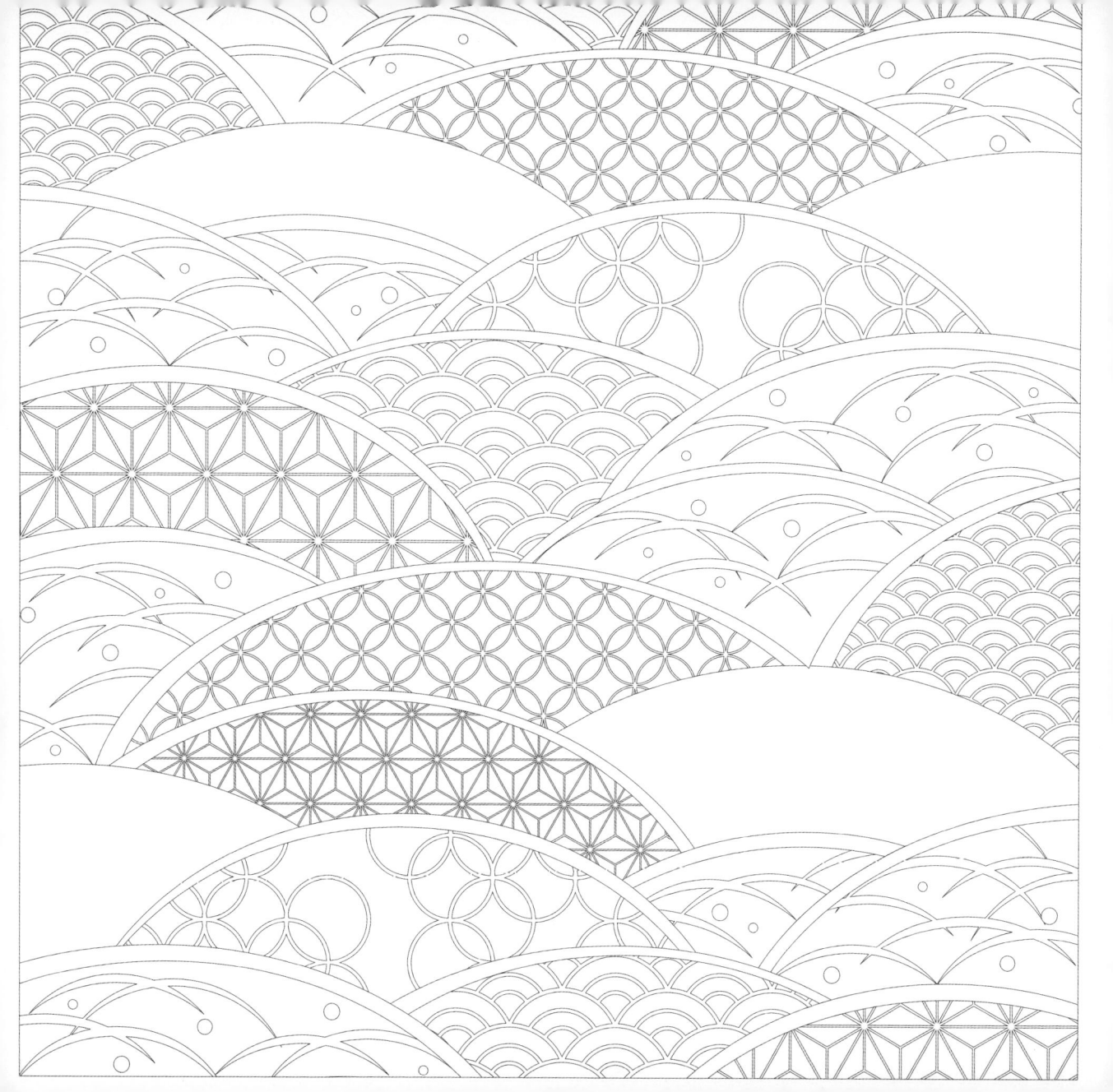

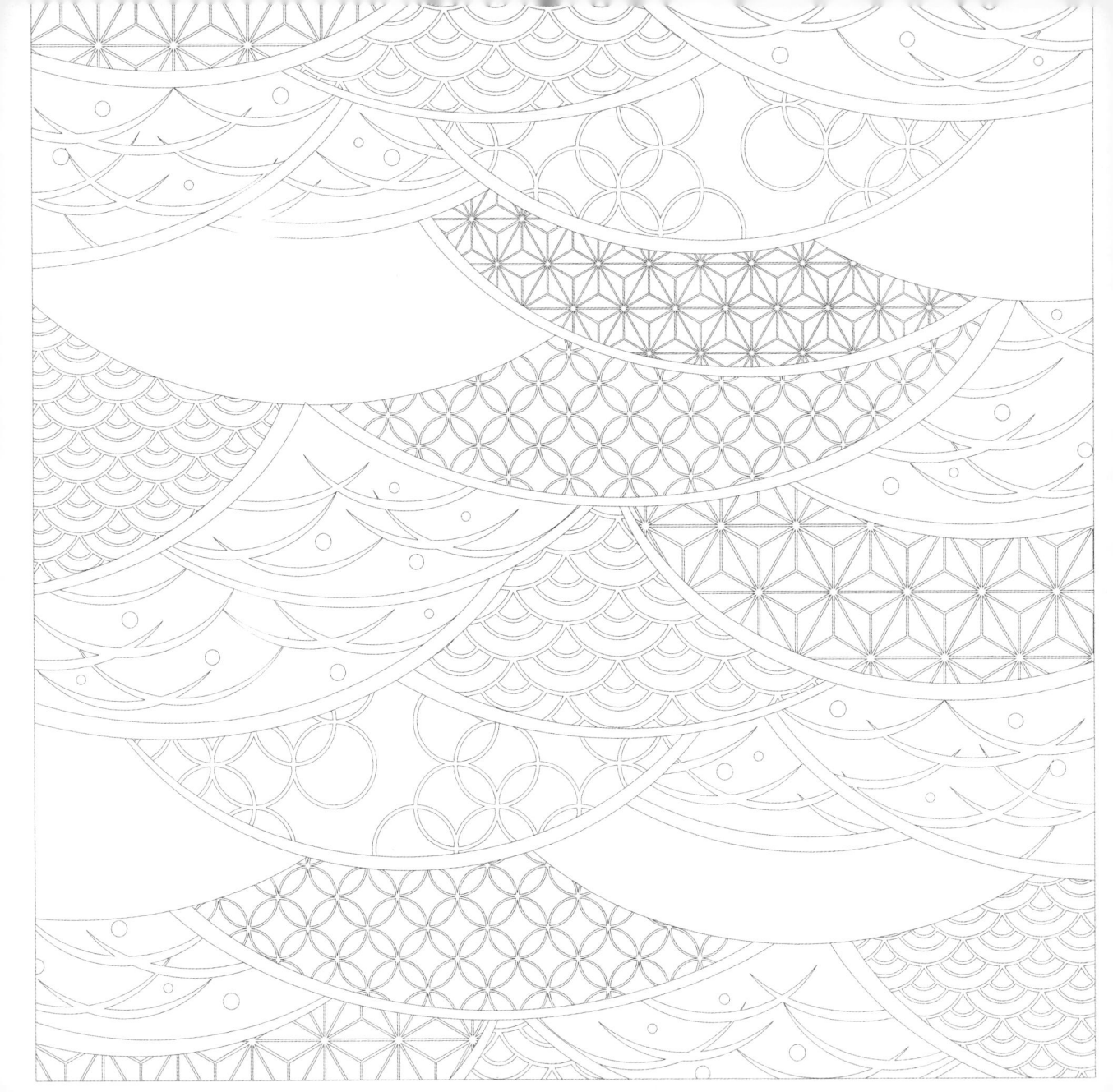

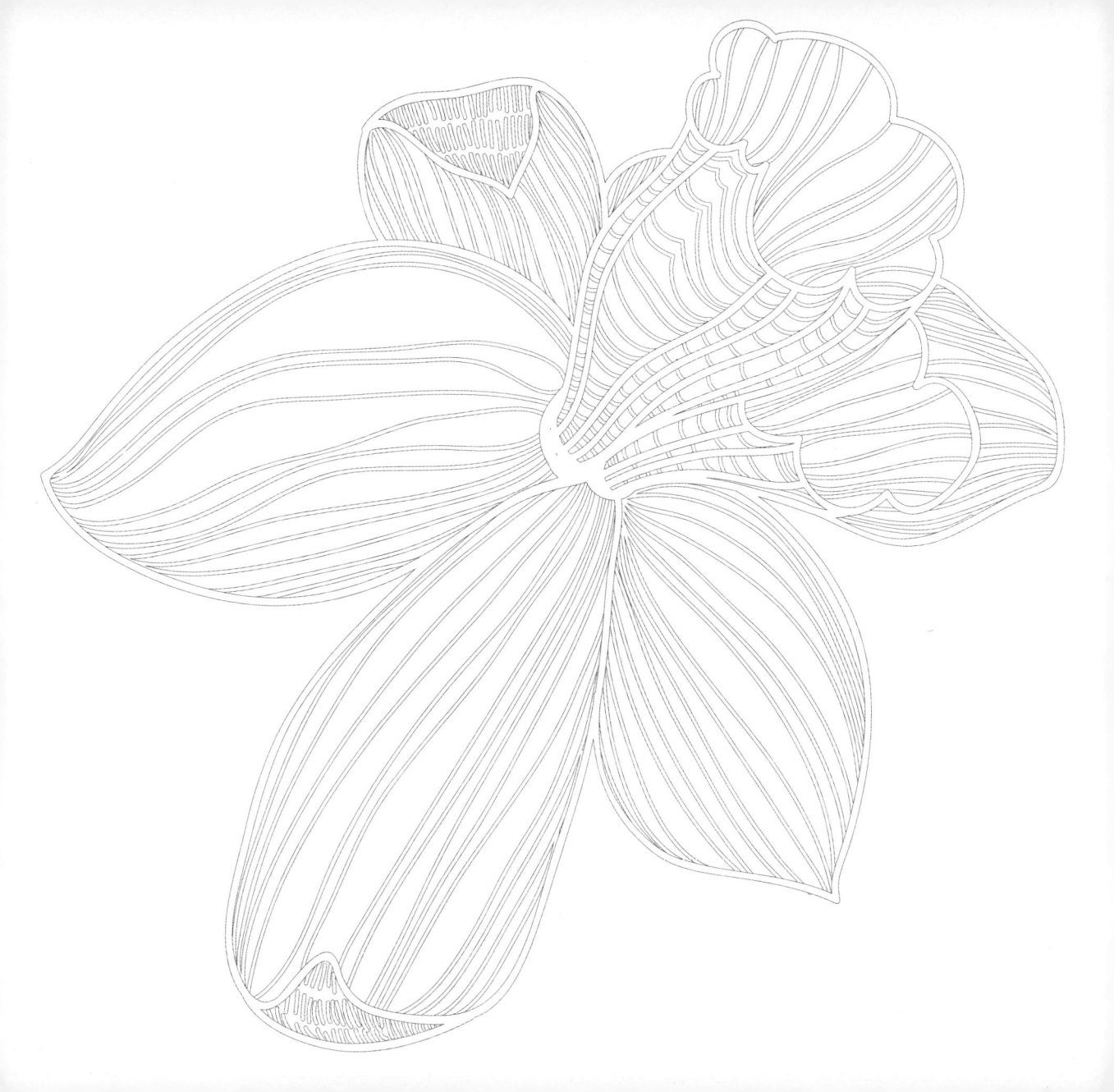

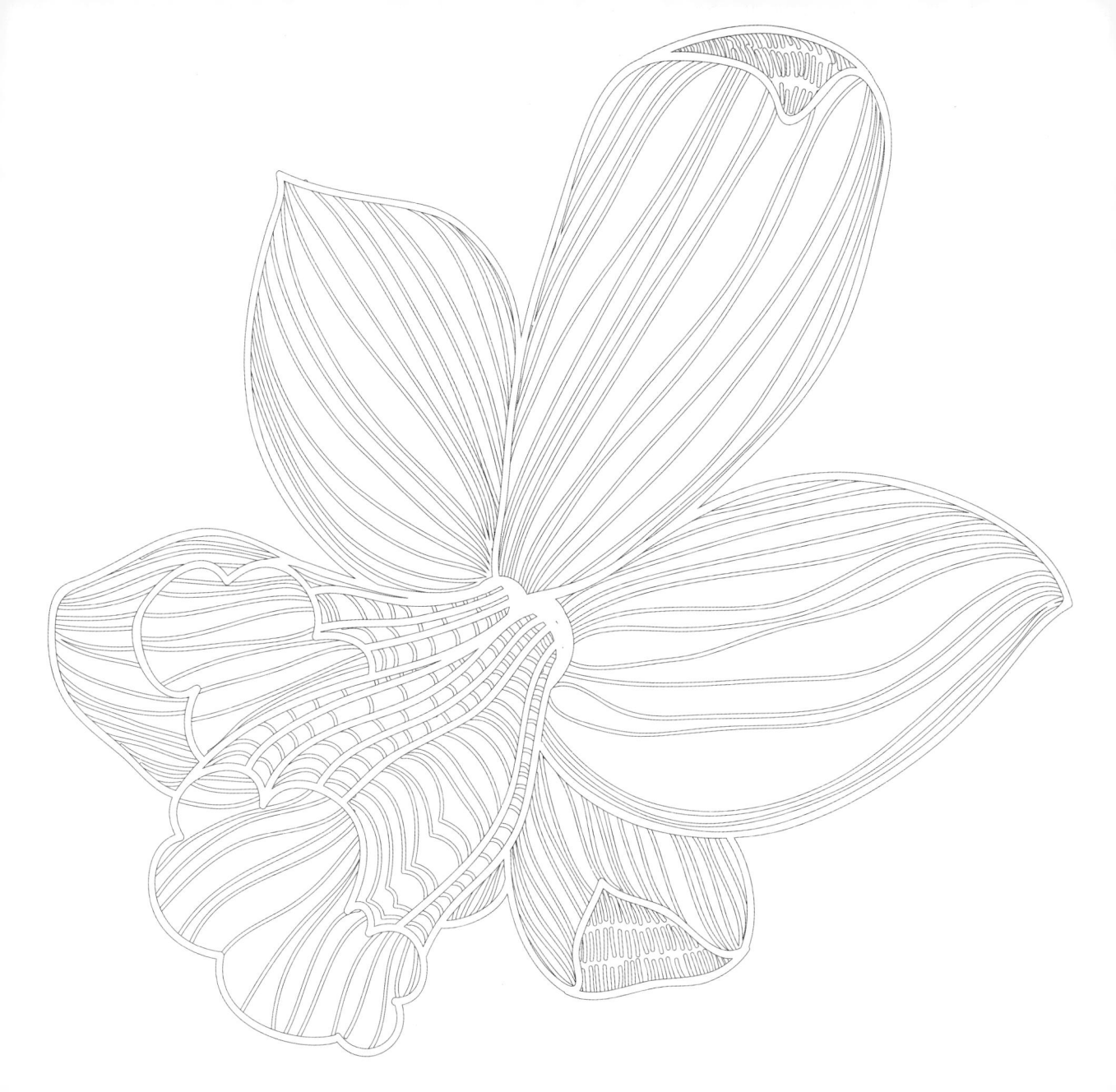

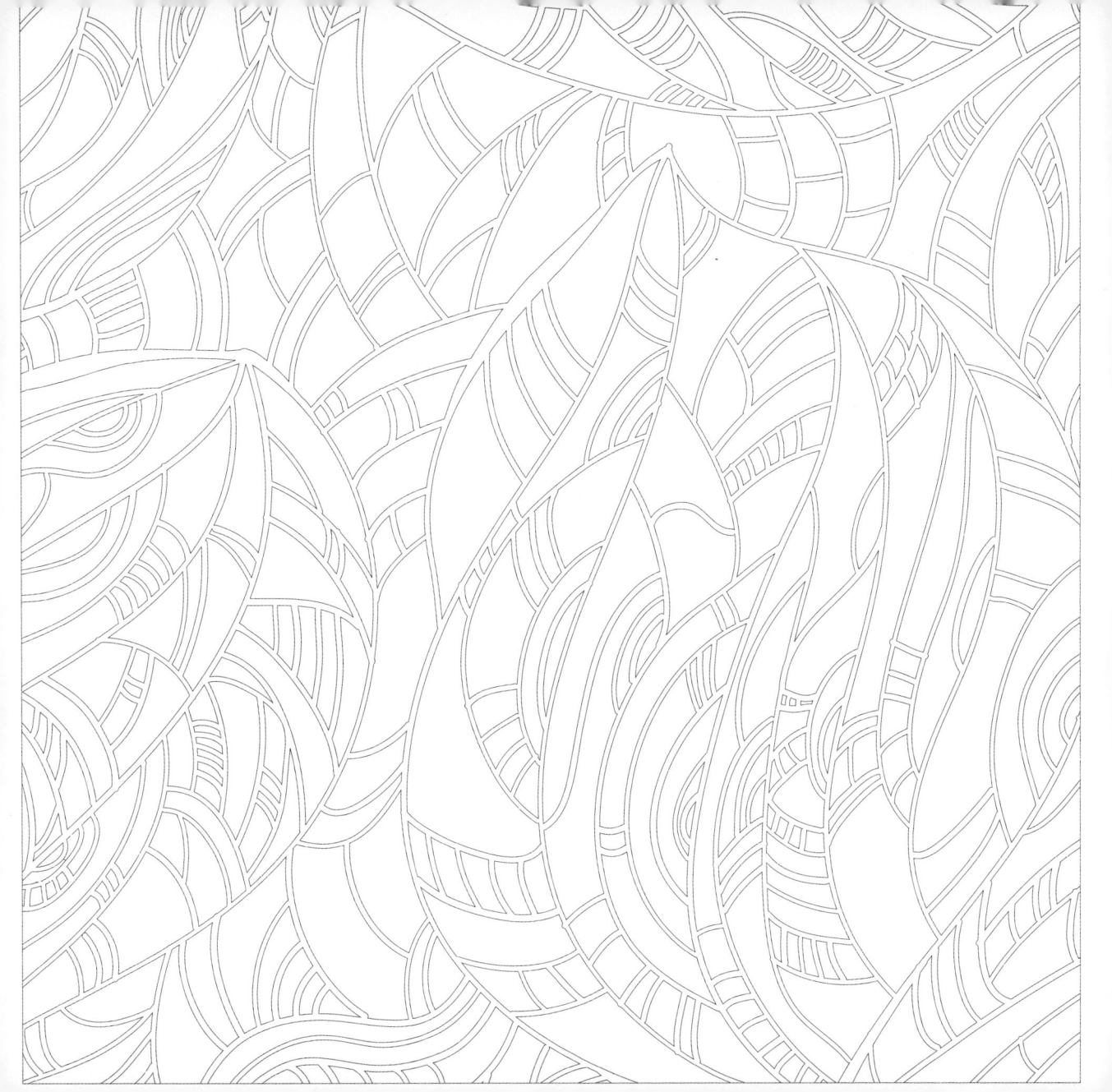

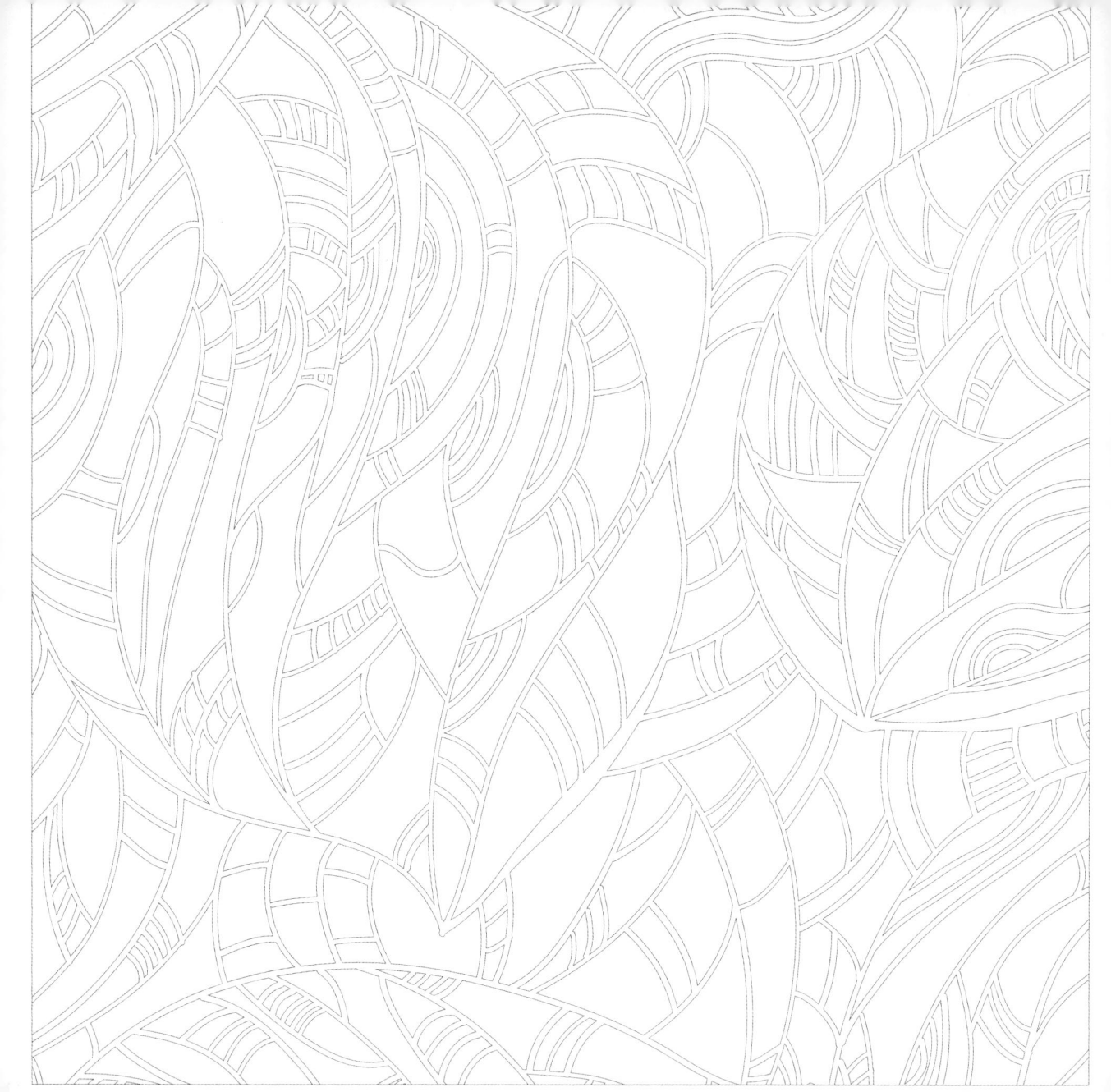

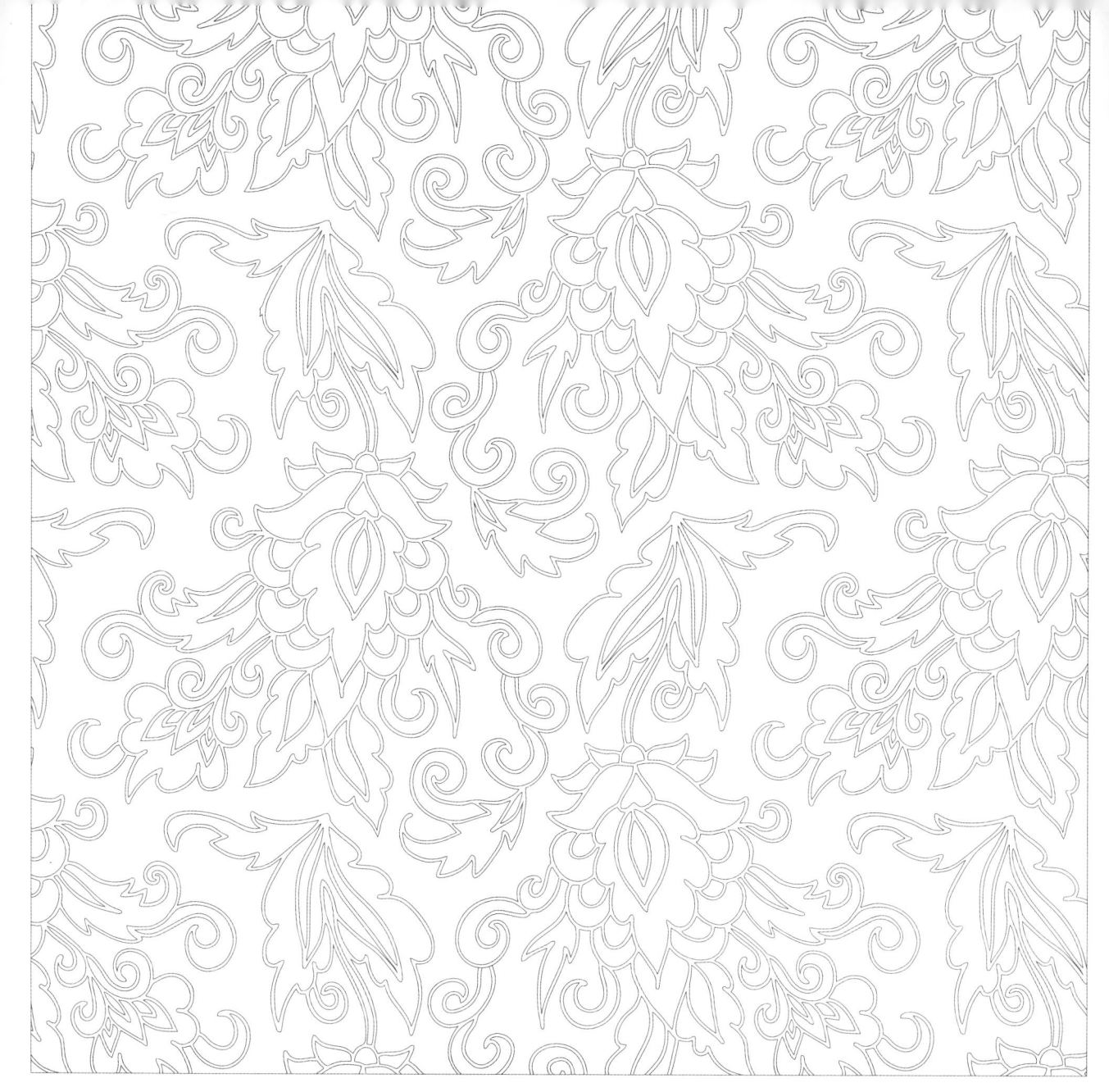

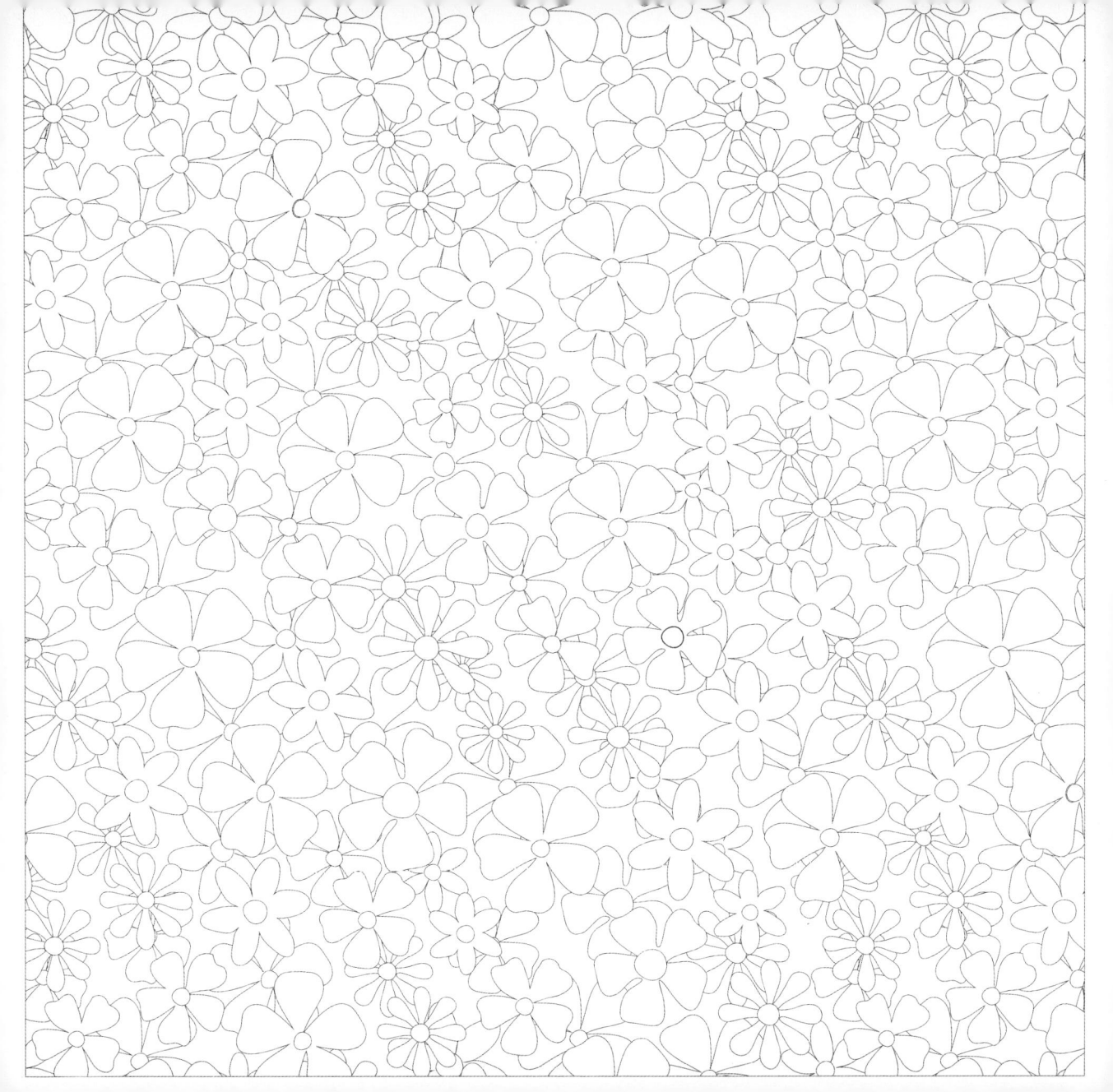

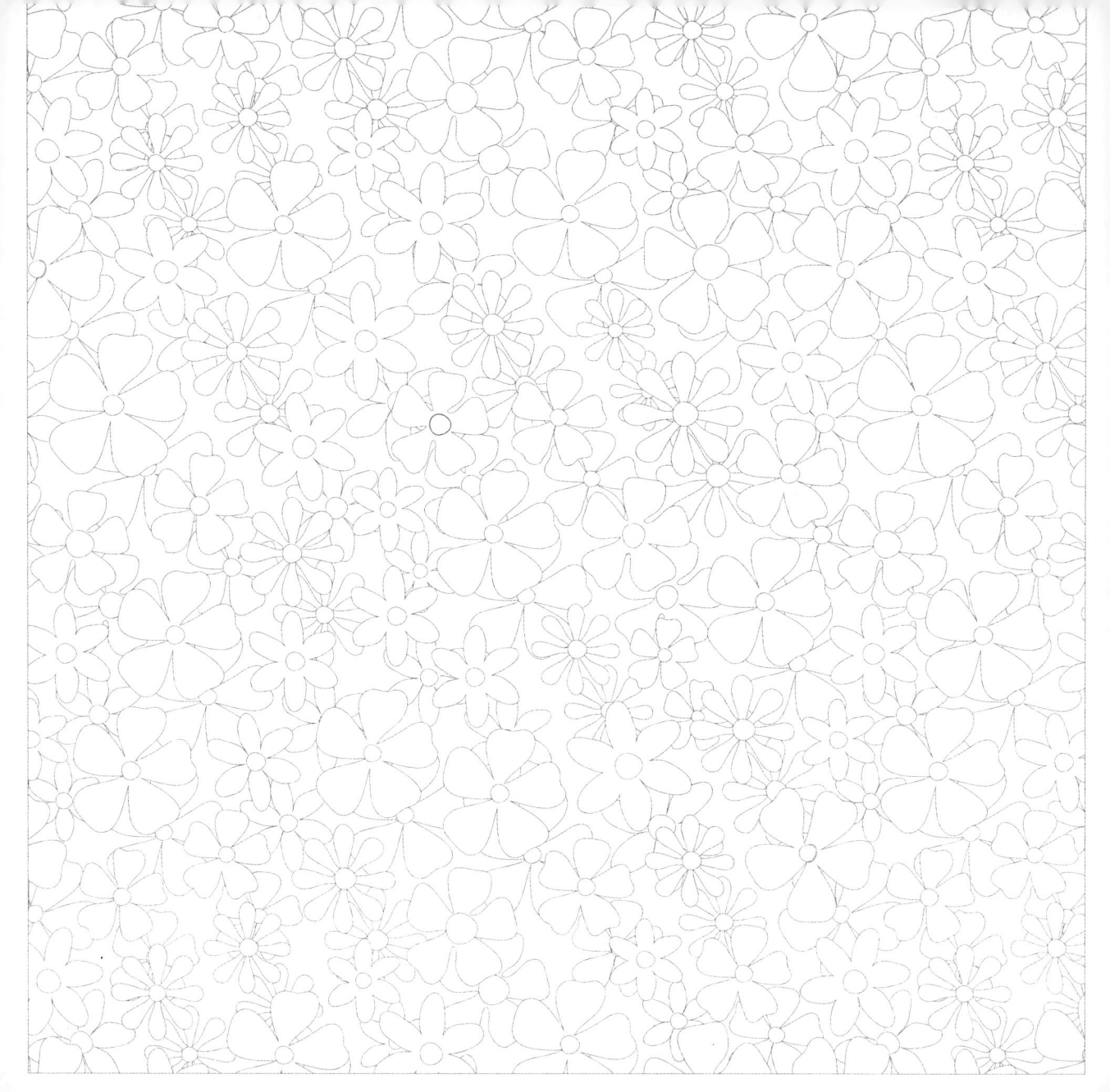

love

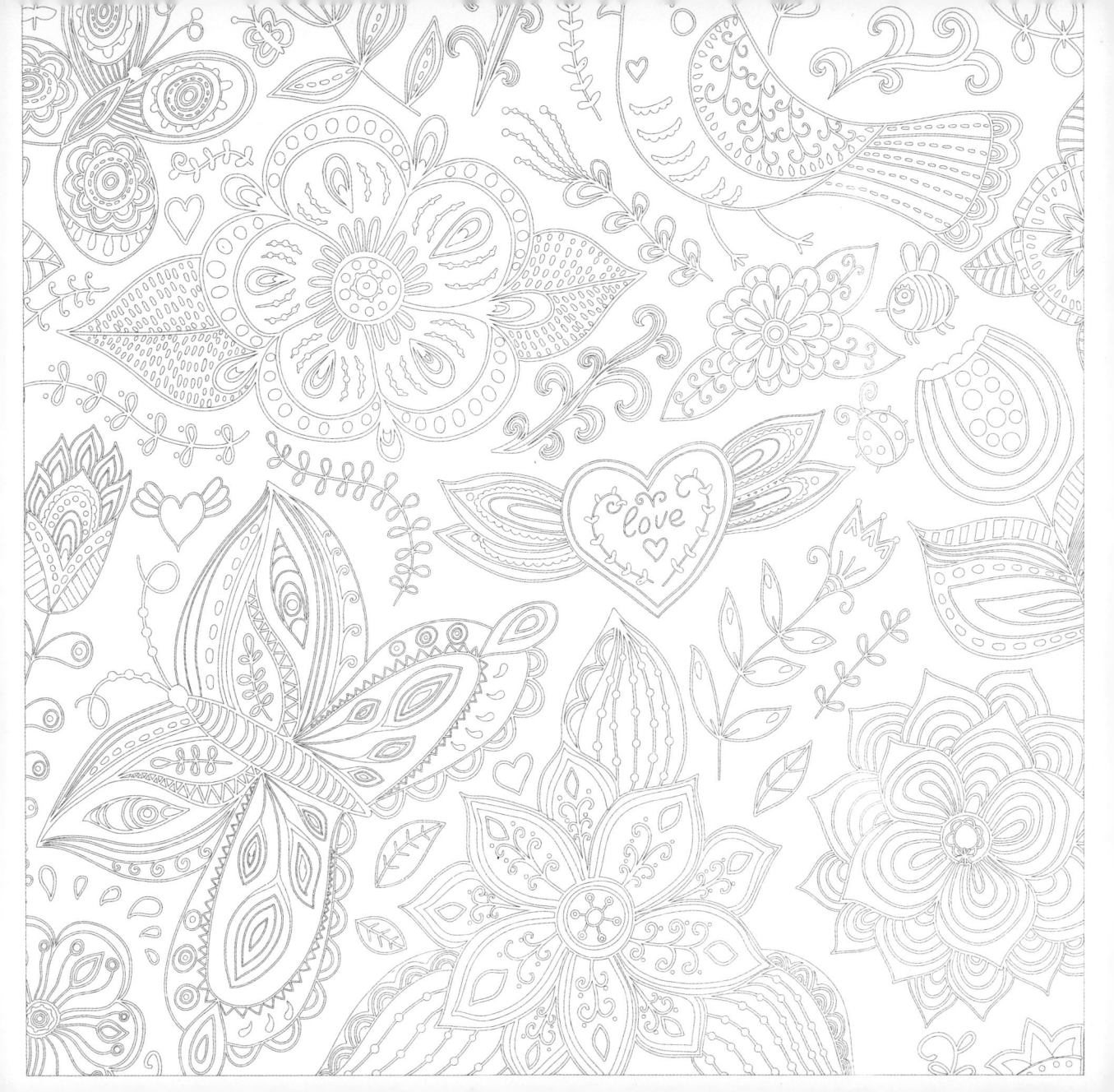

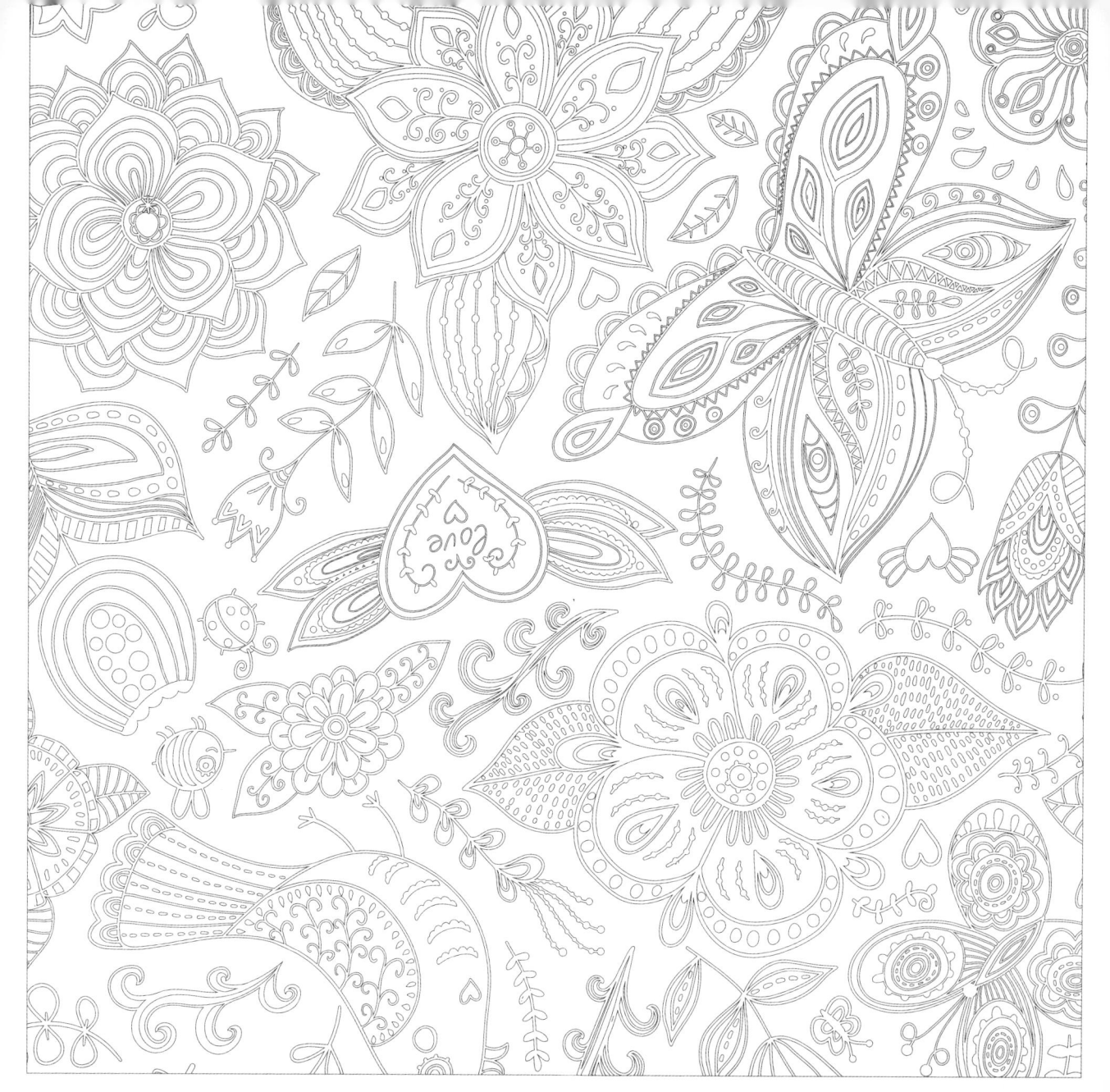

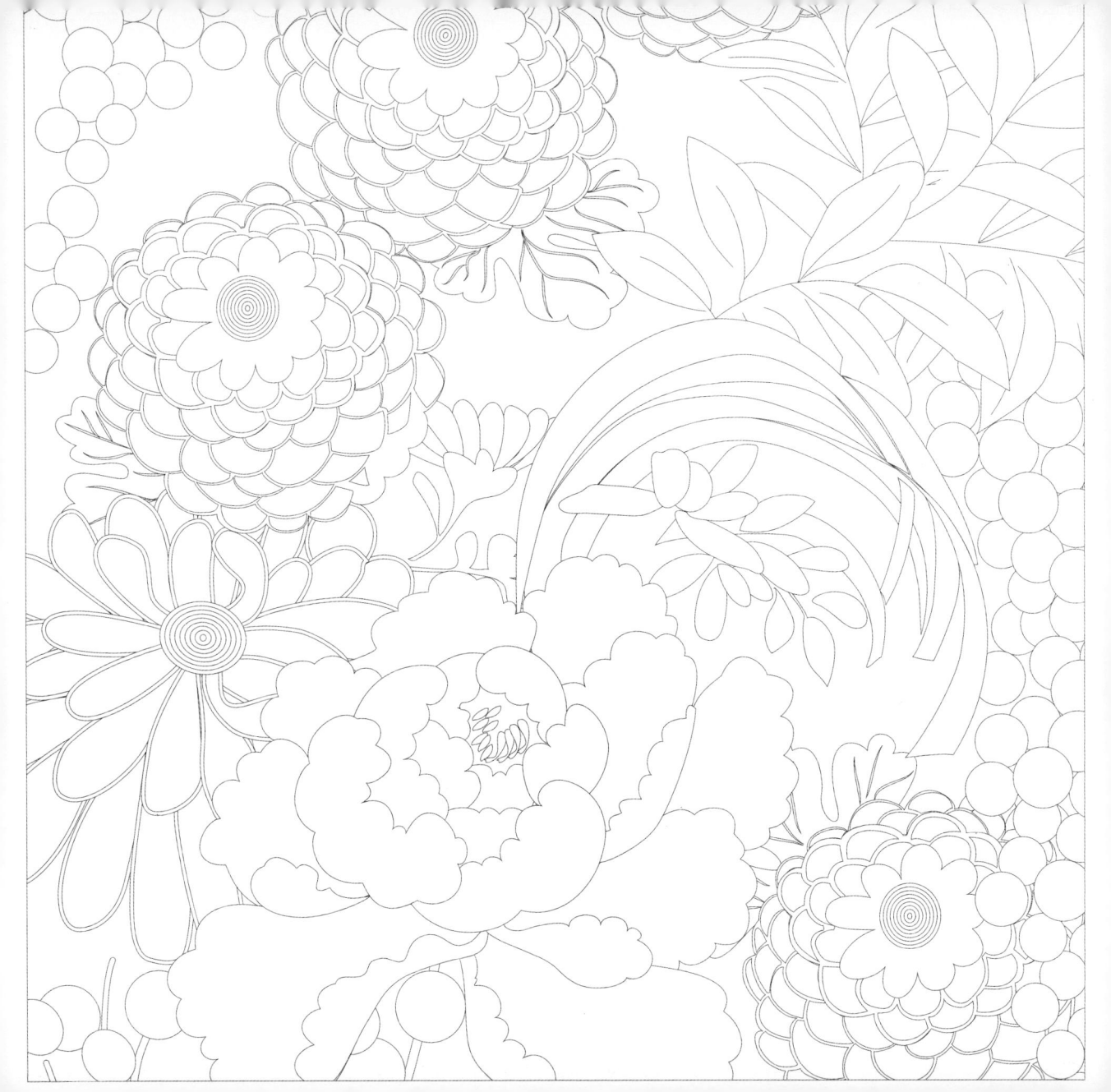

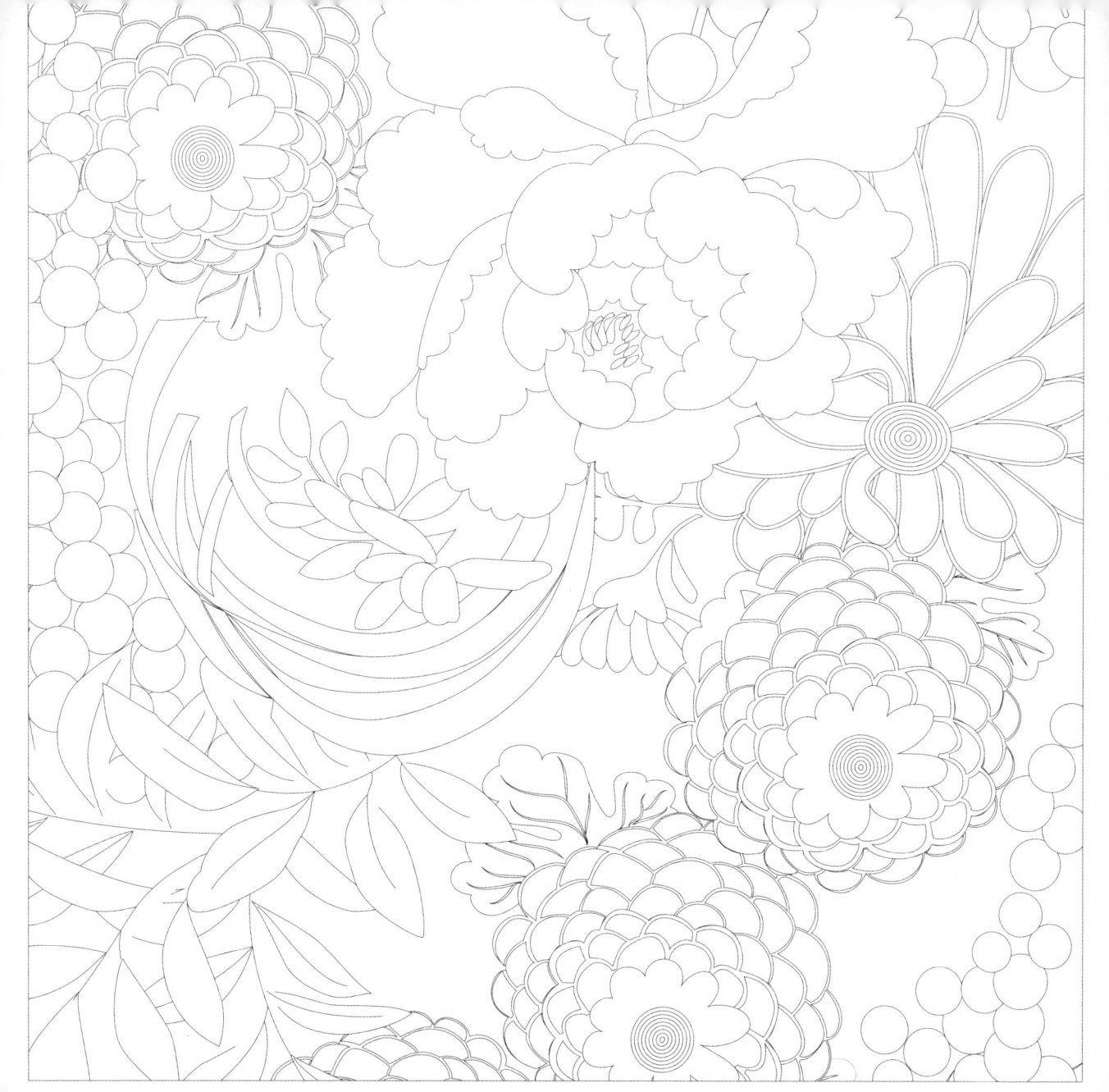

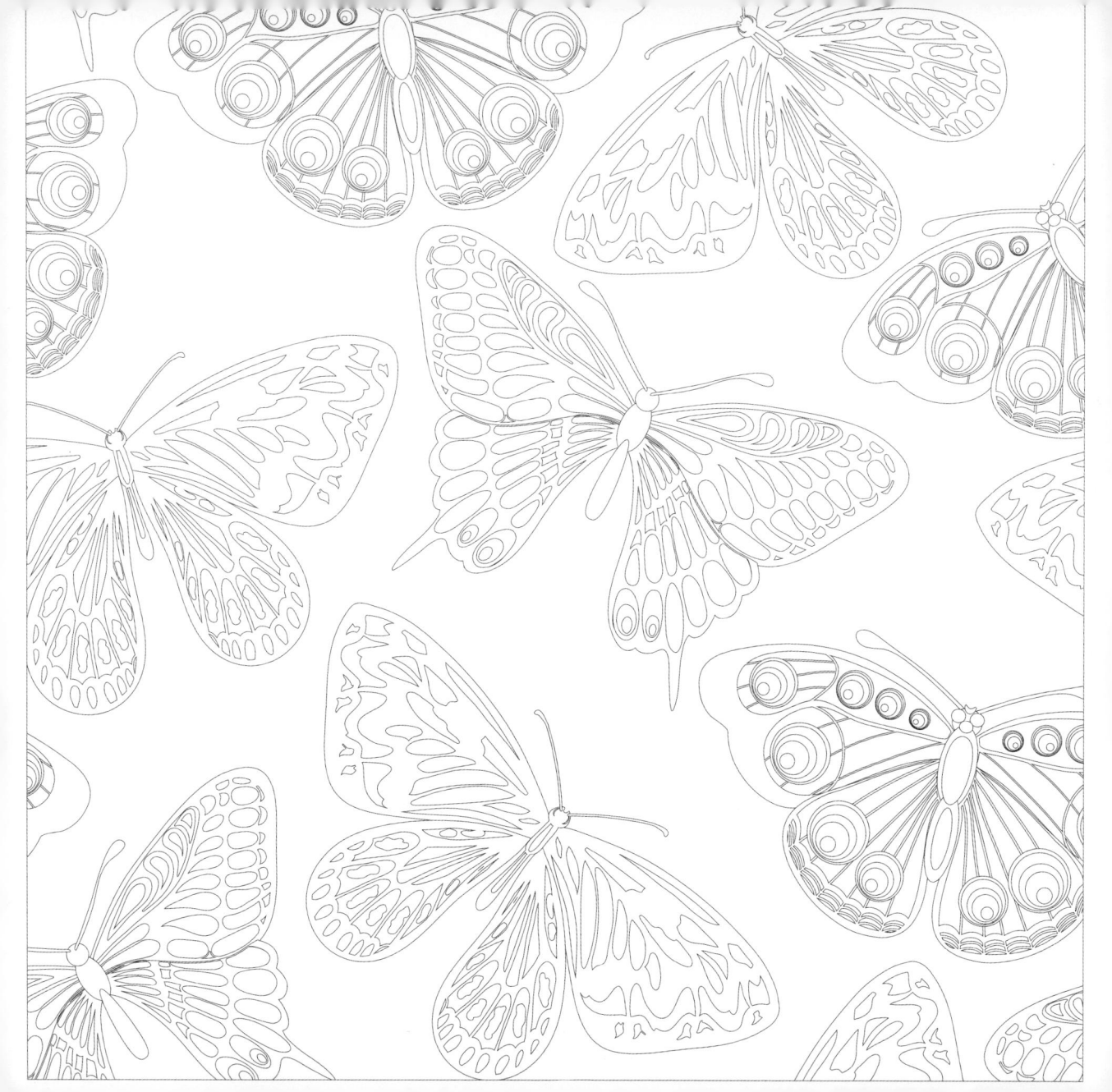

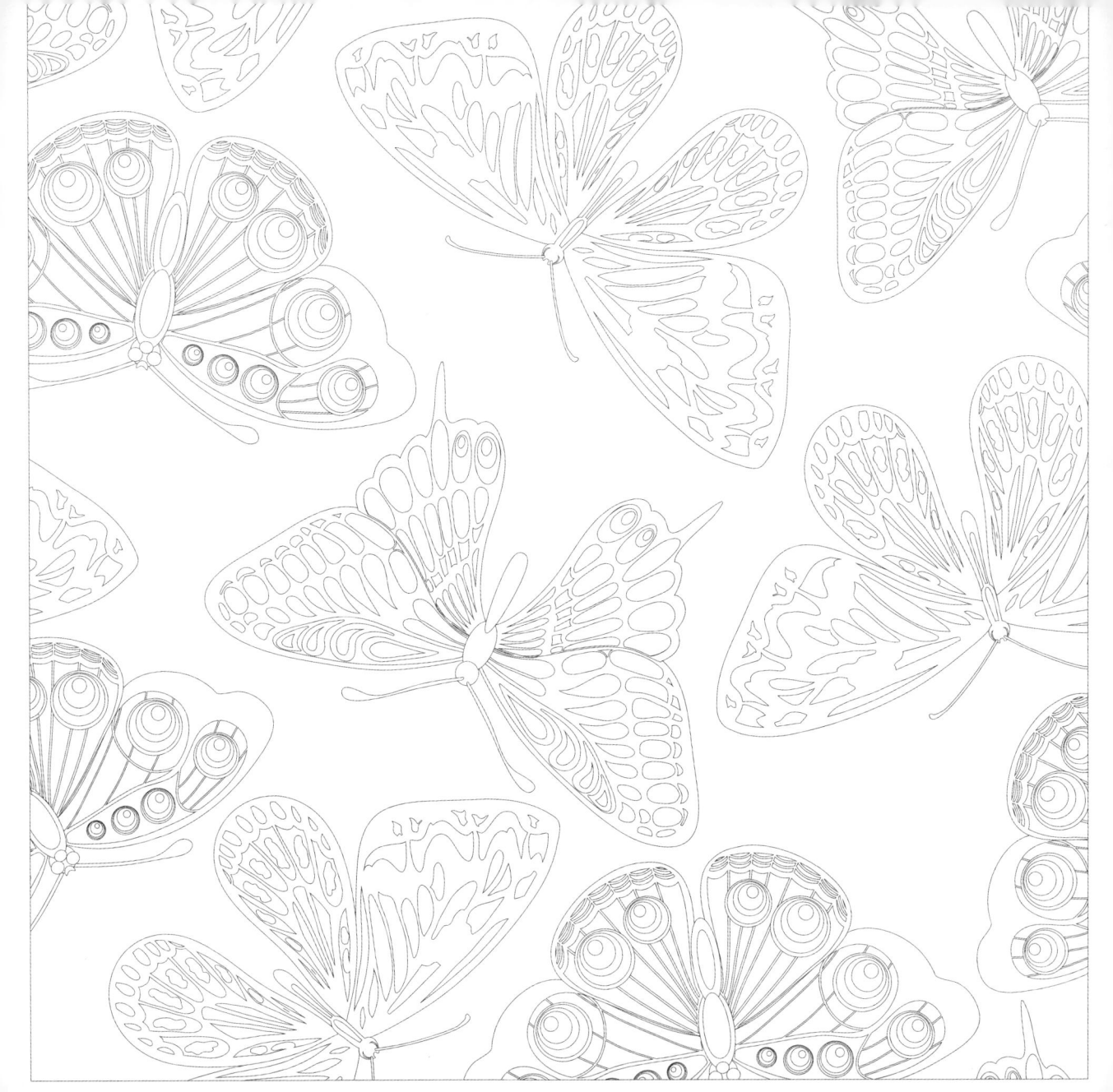

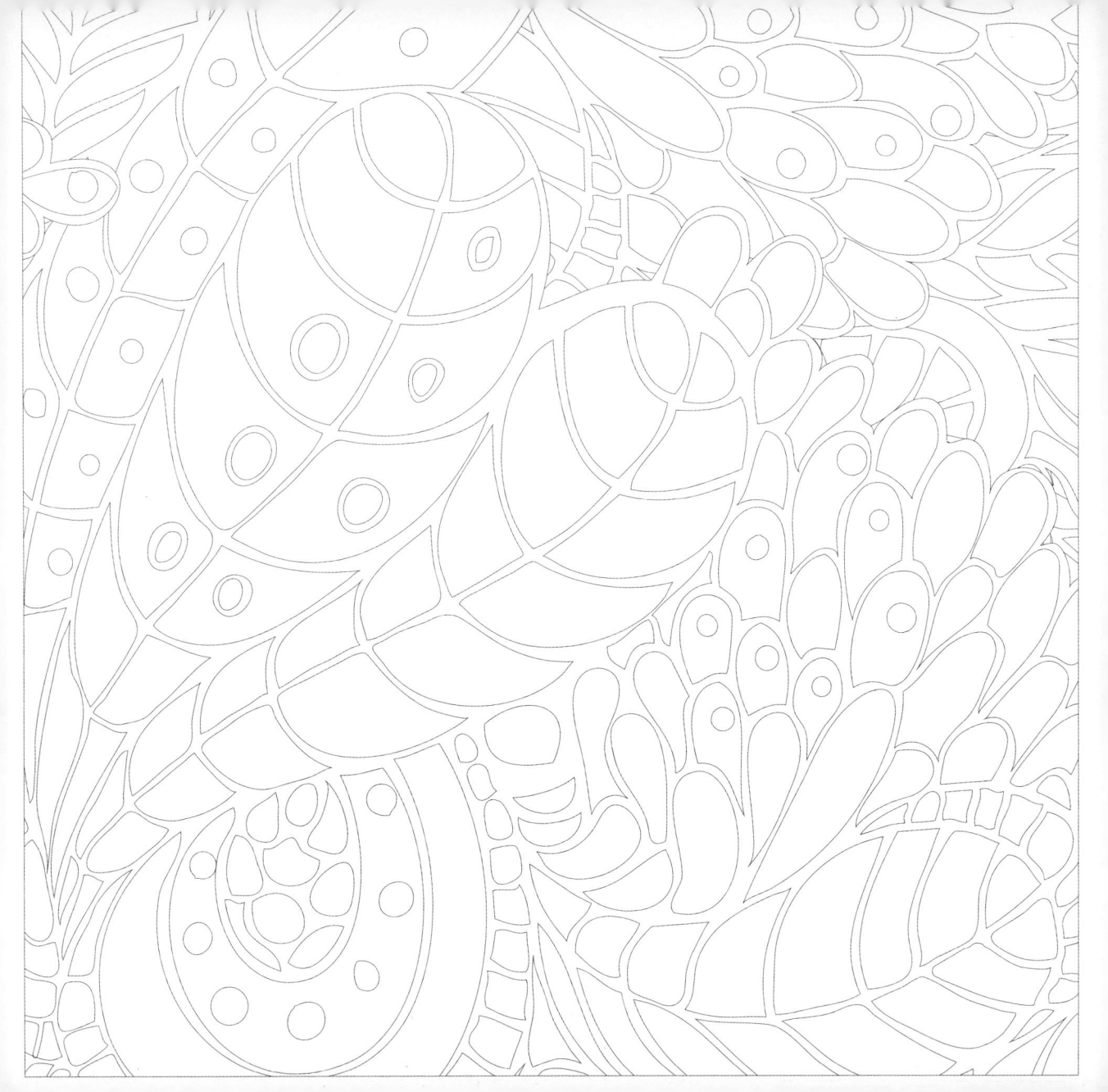

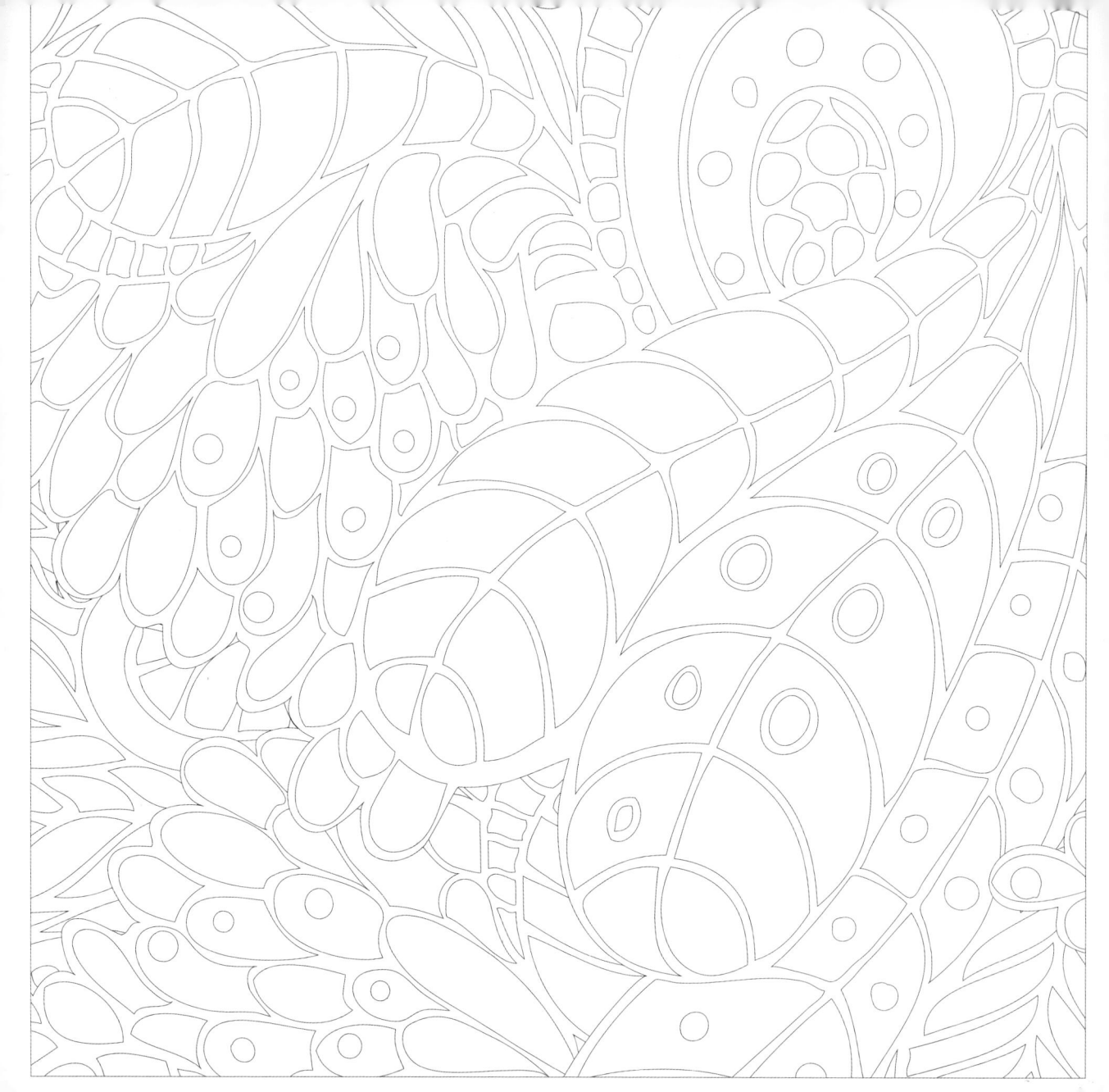

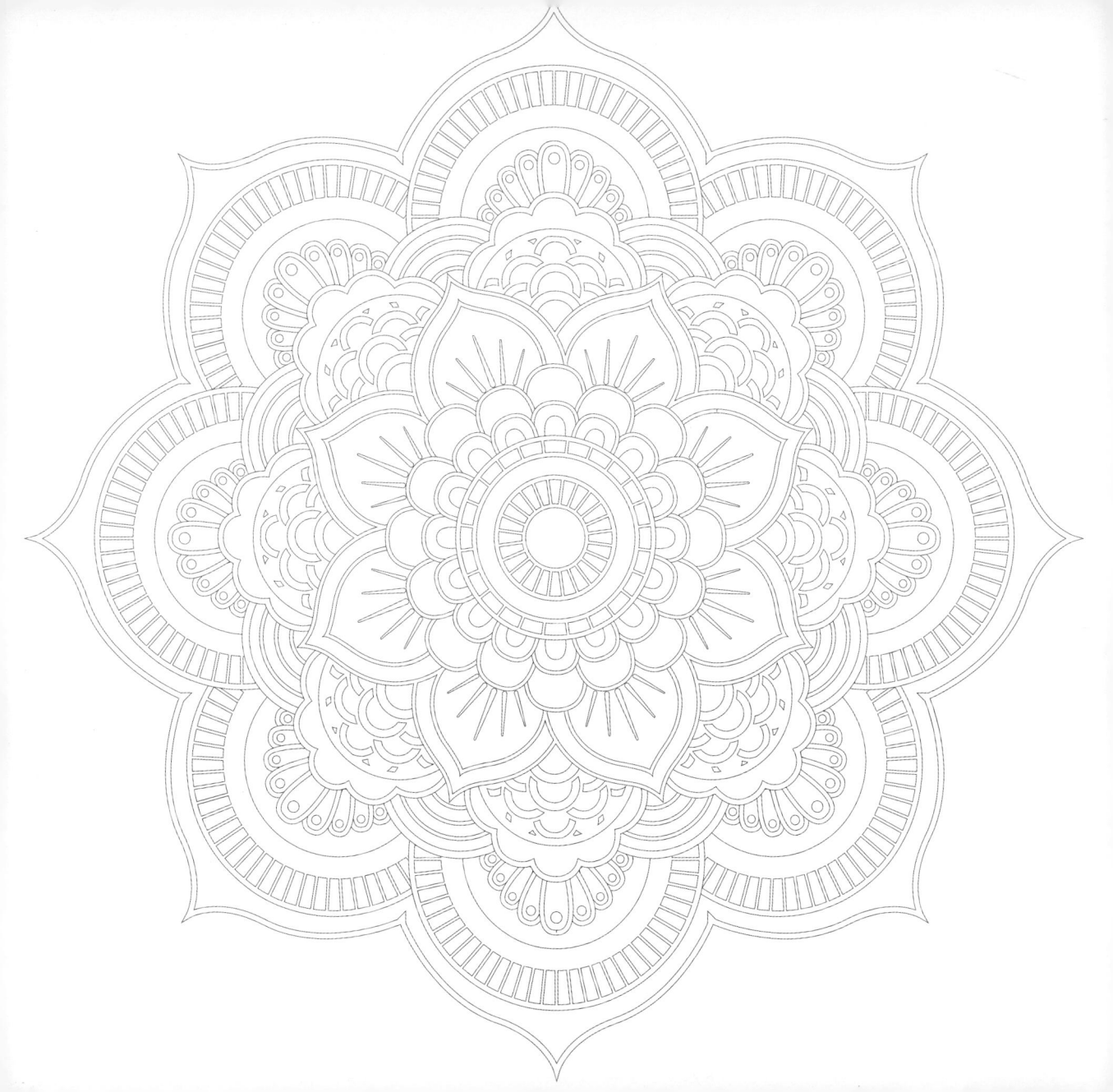

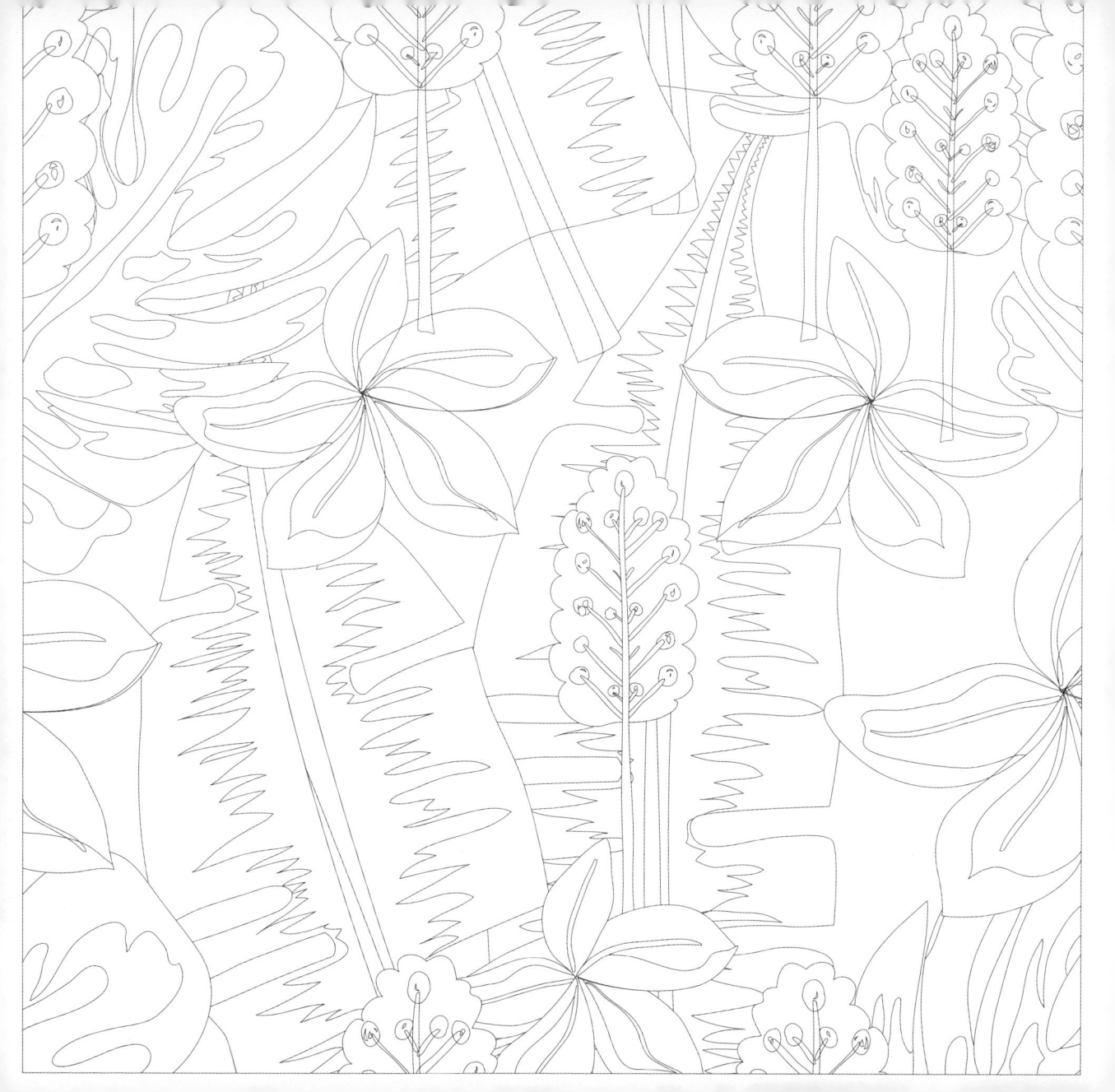

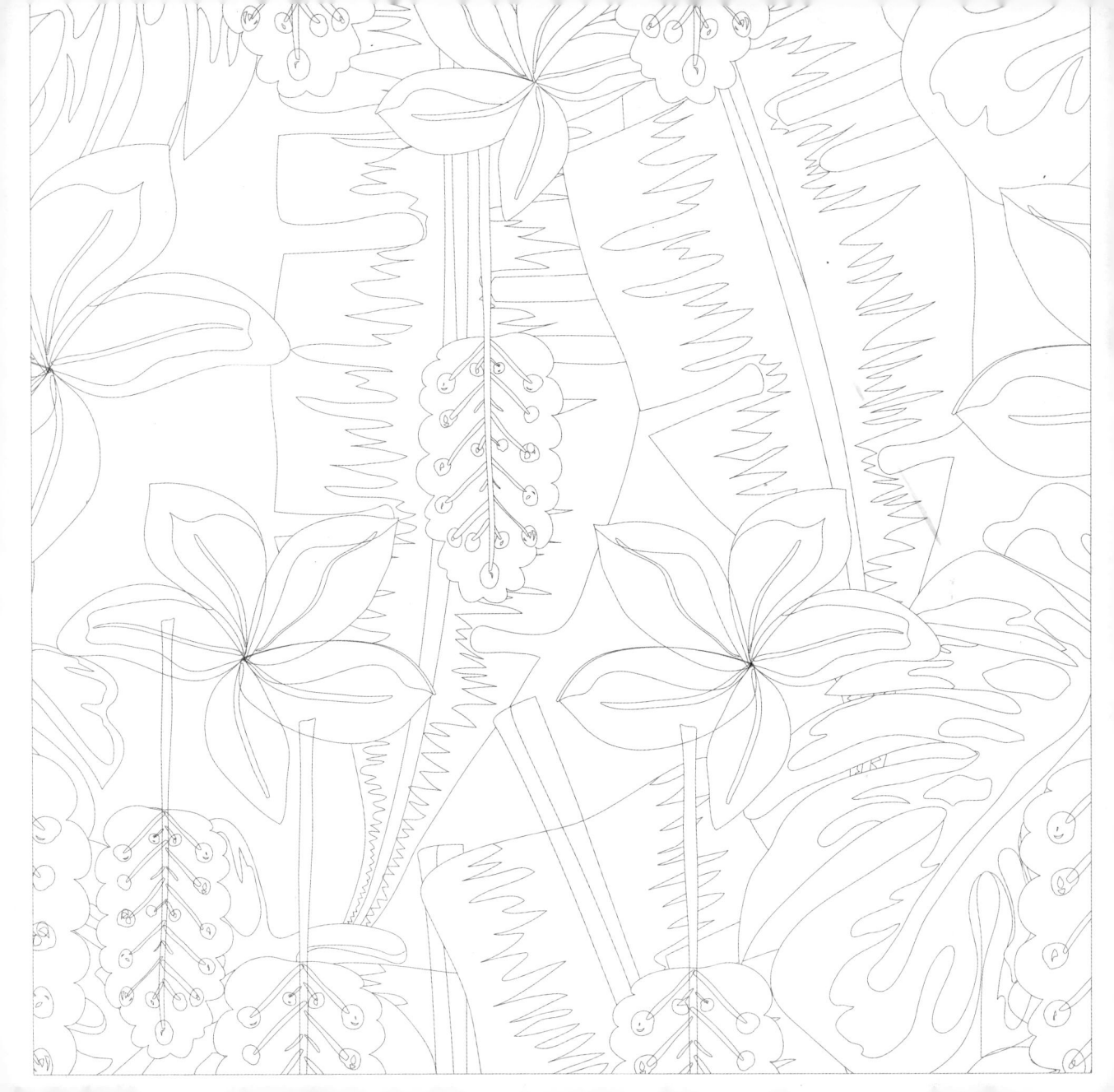